Healing Gone Wrong

Healing Done Right

Healing Gone Wrong
Healing Done Right

Ray M. Schilling, MD

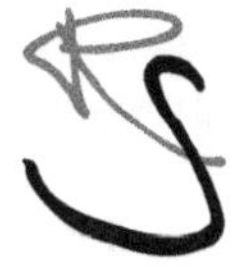

Healing Gone Wrong - ***Healing Done Right***
Ray M. Schilling, MD

Book and Cover Design by Karoline Butler

ISBN-10: 1523700904
ISBN-13: 978-1523700905
Library of Congress Control Number: 2016901564
CreateSpace Independent Publishing Platform
North Charleston, South Carolina

Dedication:

I dedicate this book to those who are willing to work on prevention in order to achieve a longer life without disabilities.

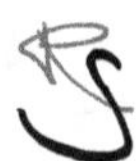

Contents

Introduction

The purpose of practicing medicine, the healing art, is to make a suffering patient better and to help cure an illness. This is what Paracelsus had in mind when he taught medical students 500 years ago. He is considered the father of modern medicine. But often in modern times the outcome of medical interventions is not what it should be. Now that I am retired, I have time to think back and reevaluate where I came from, based on what I have seen. Currently I keep two medical websites up to date and write two blogs per week, and as a result I research very closely what is going on in medicine today. In the course of this research I also come across aspects of medicine that lack common sense. The title of "Healing Gone Wrong – Healing Done Right" comes from these observations. I am hoping that we can all learn from some of the mistakes of the past. However, we will also see that enough is going wrong in modern medicine now, and this book will deal with these aspects in detail.

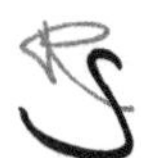

My Background

I completed my medical training and my internship in a traditional medical school in Germany in1972 after which I relocated to Canada and spent a few years doing cancer research at the Ontario Cancer Institute in Toronto, Ontario.

There was a brief detour where I studied for 2 ½ years more as an intern at various university hospitals of McMaster University in Hamilton, Ontario (mixed family medicine program). During this time I got introduced to the problem-oriented approach to medicine for which McMaster University is famous. I also passed the Canadian State examination in 1978, called the LMCC.

I started to practice family medicine in a small town of Southern British Columbia. My senior associate had a wealth of practical knowledge, and he was generous and happy to share his experiences with me. I understood more and more that medicine was not strictly a science, but also an art. As I looked after patients over the years I noticed that very frequently there was a common denominator to the problems of the aging patients: first they realized to their dismay that they had a lack of energy, but in the wake of this various illnesses deprived them of their "golden years". Ailments like arthritis, heart disease, diabetes, lung disease and cancer took center stage.

Prevention had not yet become the word that was in everybody's mouth. I knew about vitamin supplements, and recommended vitamin E for heart health, which resulted in snarky remarks from some of my more conservative colleagues.

I came to the conclusion that any disease would be better prevented before it could wreak havoc with the health of a patient. Over the sixteen years of my family practice in Langley, B.C. I believed in prevention. I encouraged my patients to do everything that was known at the time to prevent obesity, high blood pressure and manage stress through relaxation techniques. It was gratifying to see success! In many instances patients were able to get back to normal blood pressure readings or managed to successfully combat diabetes with dietary and other lifestyle changes.

In the second phase of my career I dealt with occupational medicine. It was often obvious how problematic lifestyles paved the way to arthritic changes and back problems. In these cases prevention was too late, and the only choice was conventional curative medicine like anti-arthritic medications and eventually surgical joint replacements. I was still involved in treating patients in a walk-in clinic setting on the side. However, in that setting there was a time constraint in examining and talking to patients. Yet it was very clear that patients had questions that could not be dealt with in a 5 to 10 minute visit. My next project in 2002 was the creation of two medical websites that would be accessible to everybody and give medical information in everyday language. This is how www.nethealthbook.com got started, and soon after I started writing also a medical blog, www.askdrray.com. During all the years of practicing medicine I found out more about medical research at conferences for continuing medical education. But there were also new pathways in medicine. A small group of physicians had founded the A4M, the American Academy of Anti Aging Medicine. The number of A4M members increased dramatically over the years to 26,000 physicians in 2013. I joined them as a member in 2008. I became curious about the conferences that were organized by A4M and have since attended an A4M conference in Las Vegas every year as will become evident to you when you read the blogs of www.askdrray.com.

Since 2010 when I turned 65 I have been retired. I continue to update my two medical websites, published my first book "A Survivor's Guide to Successful Aging" in 2014 and am publishing now this book "Healing Gone Wrong - Healing Done Right".

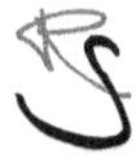

About This Book

Medical errors, false diagnoses and wrong treatments are nothing new in the history of medicine. It happened in the past, and it is happening now.

Chapter 1 describes that famous people like President Kennedy, Elvis Presley, Churchill, Beethoven or more recently Michael Jackson have something in common: all of them suffered the consequences of blatant medical mistakes. In Beethoven's time lead containing salves to plug the drainage holes from removing fluid from his abdomen caused lead poisoning. In this chapter I review also how the illnesses of the above-mentioned celebrities were treated, but then ask the question: "What could have been done better to prevent some of the disastrous treatment outcomes?"

Chapter 2 deals with how modern drugs seem to come and go. We learn that twenty-first century medications that are touted as the latest therapeutic agents are having their potentially deadly consequences too: COX-2 inhibitors, the second generation of "improved" arthritis drugs cause strokes and heart attacks! Your doctor may still prescribe some of these dangerous drugs for arthritis now.

Chapter 3 deals with the fact that medical treatments for people's diseases may be inappropriate when the doctor treats only symptoms, but nothing is done about the causes of their illnesses. This is a scary thought.

Chapter 4 asks the question whether we could learn something from these poor health outcomes in the past, so that we will be able to prevent any disastrous outcomes pertaining to our own health care in the present and future. As we will see, the problem today is still the same as it was in the past, namely that many physicians still like to treat symptoms instead of the underlying cause of an illness. Even though Big Pharma has the seducing concept of a pill for every ill, it is not always in your best interest, when these medications have a slew of side effects. "Gastric reflux" means a mouthful of stomach acid. This is a fact the suffering patient knows already! Big Pharma simply offers the patient with the symptom of gastric reflux a multitude of medications to suppress this symptom. But it is more important to dig deeper to find the reason for the illness and treat the underlying cause.

Chapter 5 concentrates on the brain and how we can keep our brains functioning optimally until a ripe old age. This review spans from prevention of head concussions to avoiding type 3 diabetes (insulin sensitivity from overconsumption of sugar).

Chapter 6 reviews what we now know about how to keep a healthy heart. Certain ingredients are necessary such as regular exercise, a healthy Mediterranean diet, supplements etc.

Chapter 7 delves into the question why healthy food intake matters. Without the right ingredients of our body fuel, the body machinery will not work properly.

Chapter 8 talks about healthy limbs, bones and joints. We are meant to stay active in our eighties and nineties and beyond. No osteoporosis, no joint replacements, no balance problems that result in falls!

Chapter 9 deals with detoxification. What do we do as we are confronted with pollution, with radiation in the environment and poisons in our daily food? A combination of organic foods, intravenous chelation treatments and taking supplements can help us in that regard.

Chapter 10 deals with reducing the impact of cancer in our lives. A lot of facts have come out in the past 10 years telling us that reduction of sugar and starchy food intake reduces cancer. Curcumin, resveratrol and vitamin D3 supplements also reduce cancer rates as does exercise and stress management. All of this is reviewed here.

Chapter 11 checks out your hormone status. Women need to avoid estrogen dominance; both sexes need to replace the hormones that are missing. By paying attention to your hormonal status and replacing the missing natural hormones with bioidentical ones, most people can add 10 to 15 years of useful, active life!

Chapter 12 is refining some of the thoughts about anti-aging. You will learn about the importance to keep your mitochondrial DNA healthy. Apart from that there are ways how to keep your telomeres longer; certain supplements that are reviewed will help. Also your lifestyle does make a big difference in how old you can turn.

Chapter 13 investigates the limits of supplements. Many supplements are useful, but you do not want to overdo it and get into toxic levels. More is not necessarily better!

Chapter 14 reviews an example of an illness, ADHD, which has been over diagnosed, has been neglected and has been over treated with dangerous drugs. An alternative treatment plan is discussed.

Chapter 15 gives you a brief summary of the book.

In this book it will become evident that it is better to prevent an illness whenever possible rather than to wait for it to set in and cause disabilities or death. You heard this before: "Prevention is better than a cure" or "an ounce of prevention is better than a pound of cure". I will give an explanation, based on scientific data that there is indeed evidence to support these notions on a cellular level. The mitochondria, the energy packages within our cells, are the driving force that keep people vibrantly healthy well into their nineties. All this can only happen when the mitochondria function properly. But if the mitochondria are poisoned and malfunction, we are not looking at a person with vibrant health. Instead sixty or seventy year-olds may be confined to a wheelchair. If you want a life without disabilities, a life without major illnesses and good health to a ripe old age, you are reading the right book.

Ray M. Schilling, MD
Kelowna, BC, Canada
January 2016

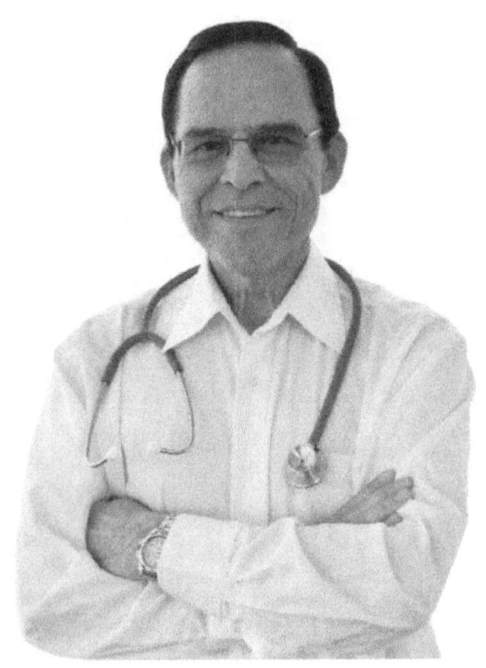

Ray M. Schilling, MD - 2016

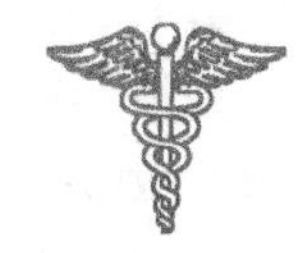

Chapter 1:

Famous Patients Failed by Medicine

Elvis Presley: overstressed and overmedicated

It was the year 1967. Elvis Presley had just turned 32, when he was totally exhausted from concert tours. This distressed him greatly, as he had to be fit to do upcoming television recordings. He needed help, and in this case he called his doctor. His regular physician was not available, so he saw Dr. Nichopoulos (Elvis called him "Dr. Nick").

This man was not only a good-looking, athletic individual, but also a personable fellow and a very good listener. Elvis liked him right away. But Dr. Nick had some other means than just listening skills. He gave his patient a good dose of Dexedrine to pep him up. No wonder that Elvis was up to anything after that: Dexedrine is an amphetamine, and amphetamines have the quality to make anybody hyper. The good doctor also wanted to make sure that the patient would be able to have a restful sleep after his strenuous

work. A prescription for Placidyl- a sleeping pill- was also issued, and to make really sure that the stimulating effects of amphetamines would be knocked out, he gave him some Seconal as well! Seconal is a barbiturate that produces not only a deep sleep, but also a solid hangover. Today any physician playing with a drug cocktail like that would lose his license. For a while things went well, but about one year later Elvis needed the help of Dr. Nick again. He suffered from an acute eye condition (uveitis) and Dr. Nick arranged for an ophthalmologist who saw him on an urgent basis. As the pain in the eye was so severe, that the patient was extremely uncomfortable, a strong dose of Demerol (Pethidine) was given intravenously and subsequently cortisone was injected directly into his affected eye. Within a day his symptoms disappeared and the eye condition was healed. Elvis most certainly was very impressed. But we know that this was not a medical miracle! Demerol is one of the strongest pain medications that are available, and cortisone is extremely effective to bring down inflammation and swelling. Unfortunately however, Elvis was so impressed by the effects of Demerol that it became his favorite pain medication. Elvis was worried that Dr. Nick would not give him Demerol prescriptions on the long-term, as this morphine derivative is known to be addictive, and he knew that it was a controlled drug. This did not worry him too much. He secured an alternative supply of Demerol through a physician in California. At this time prescription information between the various states was not easily communicated. This was before computers and e-mail, and California was far away. On October 15, 1973, five days after his divorce from his wife Priscilla, Elvis was brought to a hospital in a comatose condition. Physicians noted that his whole body was covered with needle marks and skin hemorrhages (hematomas) from drug injections. He also suffered from liver enlargement and from intestinal

obstruction. Over the few years Elvis had gained a lot of weightfromovereating.Whenhismedicationsweresearched at the ranch, there were several prescription sleeping pills (barbiturates, benzodiazepines) that had been ordered by Dr. Nick. Following this serious crisis Elvis recovered, but not all was well. His lifestyle was as disastrous as before, and overeating was part of it. He was craving foods rich in calories, such as sweets and fatty foods. Dietary advice from his doctor was falling on deaf ears. For breakfast he liked to eat three double cheeseburgers with half a pound of hash browns. Dr. Nick did not recognize that his patient had side effects from all of the prescription drugs and that the addiction problem was part of this. Realizing that he could not detoxify Elvis, Dr. Nick opted to switch Elvis to less addictive medications. The food addictions were treated as a separate problem with various diet plans. As all of them failed, he was enrolled in a diet clinic, where he could drink as much papaya juice as he wanted. When he left the clinic he had gained 13 more pounds!

At age 40 a typical day for Elvis went like this: he would get up in the early afternoon; he got his first dose of amphetamines to get him going. 1 or 2 hours later he received an injection of Halotestin (fluoxymesterone), a synthetic testosterone injection. This was to compensate for a lack of sex drive as a result of his use of sleeping pills. If he felt dizzy from the side effects of Halotestin, another medication was given for that. In the evening he received another dose of amphetamine to prepare his energies for the evening concert. He also received a diuretic for urine production and medication to stimulate his bowels to overcome the sluggishness of his bowels. Constipation is a well-known side effect of the pain medications! One hour before the show Dr. Nick gave Elvis a combination of codeine and caffeine. He needed to be dynamic and fired up to perform and reap waves of applause, but in reality it was like another whip for a tired horse. After the show Elvis' system did not receive the rest it needed, but more medications. He received an antidepressant, some Inderal (a beta blocker) to lower his blood pressure, and an antihistamine to settle his irritated airways. Since he probably was too wound up to sleep, he also received a sleeping pill of his choice. The entire assortment is a hair-raising mix of pills!

Between 1975 and 1977 Dr. Nick had ordered more than 18,000 doses of amphetamines, along with medications against anxiety and painkillers. In the last 7 months of his life Elvis had swallowed more than 5000 tablets, which had been prescribed by Dr. Nick and three other health professionals (Dr. Elias Ghanem, Dr. Max Shapiro and Dr. Lester Hofman). Elvis died in a coma on August 16, 1977 at the age of 42. First the news was disseminated that Elvis would have died of a heart arrhythmia. However, later as details of the autopsy report leaked out it became clear that Elvis had died from the toxic effects of multiple drugs (Zittlau, 2009).

What went wrong with Elvis Presley?

With regard to Elvis Presley who died of toxic levels of amphetamines and toxic levels of medications against anxiety and painkillers, a comprehensive detox clinic program should have been able to wean him completely off these drugs. A vigorous exercise program would have created enough endorphins for the singer to feel good and strong about himself. People with addictive personalities and the associated psychological

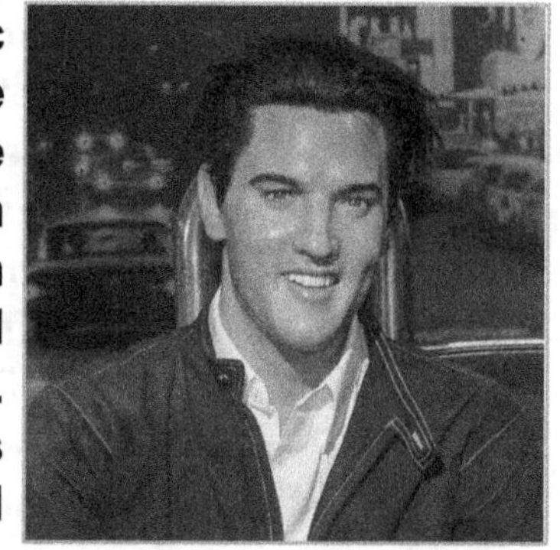

problems would also have benefitted from psychotherapy. But we also know that frequently rehab is not effective. As a result we do not know how Elvis would have responded. Like many of those patients he might not have followed through! Nowadays, saliva hormone tests or blood hormone tests would have given more accurate information about his hormone levels. In a male blood tests are as valuable as saliva hormone levels; free testosterone or bioavailable testosterone levels would have given the health care giver the information needed to judge whether a man is deficient in testosterone or not. If there were any deficiencies, these could have been addressed with bioidentical hormone replacements, not with the synthetic testosterone derivative he received. He was under a lot of stress, which can lead to adrenal gland fatigue (Wilson, 2002). In this reference text Dr. Wilson points out that cortisol levels on 4 points during the day can be measured in saliva samples and sent to a special lab. This will diagnose the degree of adrenal gland insufficiency associated with chronic stress. Chronic fatigue is often coupled with hypoglycemia, where 2 to 3 hours after a meal the patient gets hungry again. Overconsumption of sugar in fast foods, which caused him to gain weight contributed to the problem. Cutting out sugar and starchy foods would have helped Elvis to shed the pounds he wanted to lose. And he could have done it without medications and all their side effects. By bringing his hormones into balance, exercising regularly and perhaps getting some psychological counseling the King of Rock ‘n’ Roll could have lived several decades longer. However, knowing the addictive tendencies and personal problems of the artist we cannot be too sure how much longer his life would have lasted. In any event, the overuse of prescription drugs certainly contributed to his downhill course and led to his premature death.

President John F. Kennedy: pre-damaged by medicine, killed by gun shots

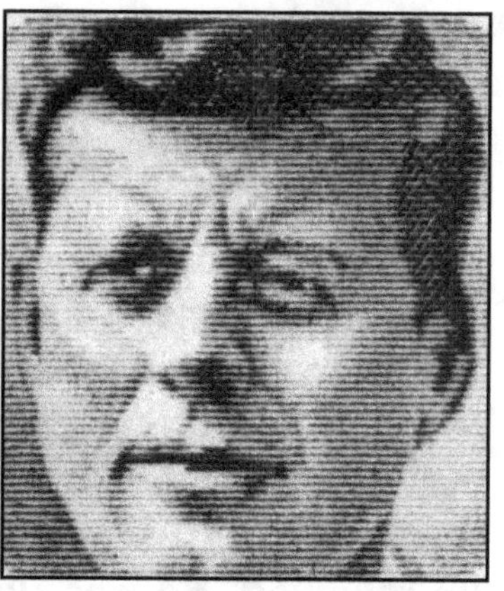

Everybody knows that President Kennedy (JFK) died from two bullet wounds on Nov. 22, 1963. Less known is his long history of chronic diseases. Despite several US hospital stays at the Mayo Clinic (1934,1938 and 1939) and another hospitalization at the Peter Bent Brigham Hospital (now part of the Brigham and Women's Hospital, Boston, MA) no explanation could be given for JFK's chronic low back pains and chronic recurrent abdominal pains or his weakness spells. In 1947 JFK collapsed in London, England while working as a newspaper correspondent and he was brought to a London clinic. There he was finally diagnosed with adrenal gland failure, also known as Addison disease. Kennedy had previously been diagnosed with inflammatory bowel disease for which he had been treated with cortisone tablets since 1937. It is known nowadays that cortisone leads to osteoporosis (brittle bones). So it does not come as a surprise that the condition of Kennedy's back had already deteriorated in 1940. He needed back surgery, and the physicians diagnosed him having osteoporosis during the surgery. The downhill spiral continued, and he was back in the hospital for more back surgery in June of 1944. However, this did not alleviate his back pains and he needed strong pain pills to be able to cope. He had entered a state of chronic pain. Contrary to his physical downhill course, his political career was soaring. JFK had become the Senator of Massachusetts in 1952. In the background more trouble was brewing. By 1954 his back

pain was so unbearable that new X-rays were ordered showing that the 5th vertebral body of the lumbar spine had melted away because of the continuous exposure to cortisone treatments. This is a condition, which is called osteonecrosis. Normally the answer would be: stop all that cortisone! But unfortunately the cortisone was necessary for his inflammatory bowel disease. As a result surgery had to come to the rescue once again. His doctors decided that he should have a steel plate inserted to bridge the gap between the 4th vertebral body and the sacral bone. There were complications following this surgery, and it took JFK a total of 6 months to recover from this surgery. All these measures did not yield beneficial results, and Kennedy's chronic back pain persisted. A new physician, Dr. Janet Travell from New York was asked for advice. Her approach was gentler than drastic surgical procedures. Small amounts of Novocain, a local anesthetic were injected intermittently into the lower back muscles that were in spasm. In the medical literature this is known as trigger point injections. Dr. Travell also found that JFK had a leg discrepancy, which caused a pelvic tilt. She prescribed an insole for his left shoe to remedy this. Dr. Travell also encouraged JFK to sit in a rocking chair for as much time as possible to relieve the muscle tension in his lower back. All this contributed to Kennedy feeling better. When President Kennedy moved into the White House in January of 1961 Dr. Travell moved in with him as his personal physician. For a period of time JFK's back was better, but the continued use of cortisone for the bowel disease caused more flare-ups of his chronic back condition. A rigid back brace was ordered by the treating physician, which was supposed to give support for the back. This was a measure popular at the time. Later it turned out that back braces should not be worn constantly as the underlying back muscles that were supposed to splint the spine were melting away from

disuse. And this is precisely what happened. JFK's back pain became so severe that another physician from New York was called in, a Dr. Max Jacobsen. He was also known under the nickname "Dr. Feelgood". The "feeling good" aspect came from very questionable treatment methods. He used dangerously high levels of amphetamines, narcotics and combined this with vitamins and human placenta. Dr. Feelgood was consulted first in September of 1960 just before the presidential debates. In May of 1961 when JFK flew to France there was a second medical advisor in the plane beside Dr.Travell. Dr. Jacobsen (Dr. Feelgood) was travelling along with the rest of the advisers. He quietly administered injections of amphetamines and painkillers, which enabled the president to control his chronic back condition. Treatment had become something that had degenerated into a "fix" of drugs. During the Vienna summit in 1961 Dr. Feelgood administered amphetamines to JFK, which kept him alert, upbeat and enthusiastic. The audiences certainly were impressed with this dynamic man, but of course they could not know that he was constantly kept hyper. Between September 1960 and May 1962 Dr. Feelgood saw the president 34 times. But with any narcotics there are prescription limits! Kennedy was in pain and determined to bypass these limits. In order to have access to amphetamines, painkillers (morphine derivatives) and barbiturates as sleeping pills, he went on shopping sprees through multi-doctoring. He also took testosterone preparations to get his sex drive back, which had been knocked out by the cortisone treatments. At the end JFK gained weight from the cortisone treatments and was very susceptible to many infections. This was due to his weakened immune system that had been relentlessly bombarded with cortisone. Also, his osteoporosis had deteriorated further, and his adrenal gland insufficiency needed to be treated with Aldosterone pills and life-long

cortisone. He was painted into a corner by medications and their side effects. As he was also entrusting himself into Dr. Feelgood's drug manipulations, he had the additional medical problem of drug dependency due to amphetamines, painkillers and barbiturates. Kennedy mentioned to people close to him that he felt that he would not live long. This was a true statement, as the clock was ticking, and it would have been only a matter of time before his health problems would have led to his demise. However, JFK was able to suppress all of this knowledge during the presidential campaign and his time as the President at the White House. Although an autopsy confirmed that JFK's death was due to a shooting with two bullets, the rest of the body was not investigated. With a life-long problem with Addison disease a proper autopsy should have included an examination of the adrenal glands and other organs. President Kennedy died at the age of only 45. His body was very likely about to give out due to chronic illness and innumerable amounts of drugs, but it was two bullets that killed him first.

What went wrong with J.F. Kennedy?

The problem with John F. Kennedy was that his adrenal gland insufficiency was not diagnosed much earlier. It was responsible for the abdominal pains, fainting spells, osteoporosis and premature osteoarthritis. With his chronic recurring lower back pains and the lack of energy he was at a higher risk of falling victim to physicians who recklessly supplied him with narcotics to combat his pain and gave him amphetamines to pep him up. In his case it was Dr. Feelgood who overdosed him with assorted drugs. We learnt from reviewing the health history of Elvis Presley and of Michael Jackson that overdoses of drugs lead to death. As we all know two bullets killed JFK. Only prevention could have saved Kennedy's life by driving in

a bulletproof motorcade or in an armored vehicle. But it is everybody's guess how much longer he would have been able to survive the daily bullet hail of medications!

Winston Churchill: seemingly invincible, but health-wise frail

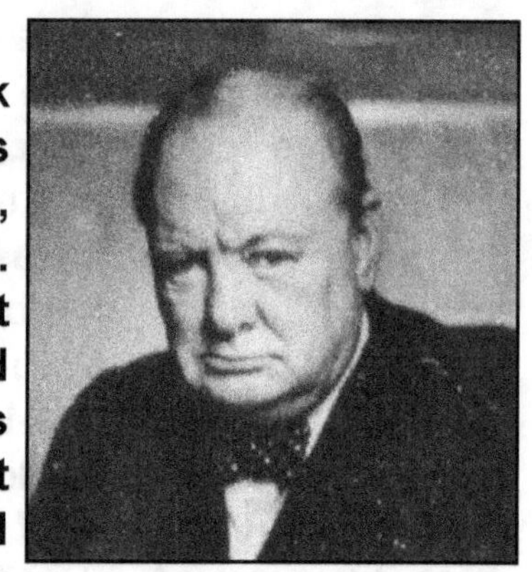

In February 1945 Yalta at the Black Sea was the location of the famous meeting between three politicians, Stalin, Roosevelt and Churchill. The Second World War had almost come to an end and Europe had to be divided. Strong decisions and energy would be needed, but it is interesting to note that all these politicians had their health issues.

Franklin Roosevelt had been paralyzed from the waist down for the past 24 years, and he had problems with his heart and circulation. The trip to Jalta was very strenuous for Franklin Roosevelt. Shortly after returning home he died of a massive stroke.

Josef Stalin was 66 years old, a chain smoker with extremely high blood pressure. He hated physicians, but there was no need for one in Yalta as he was the most energetic of the three politicians. However, later in March of 1953 Stalin collapsed, and none of the physicians present could operate the heart-lung machine as Stalin had fired his personal physician, Dr. Winogradow just three months earlier. He was the only one who would have known how to operate this medical equipment (Zittlau, 2009).

The most interesting character at the Yalta meeting was Winston Churchill. He had earned a reputation of being tough and invincible. He was able to smoke one cigar after

the other, drink whiskey, and he avoided any form of exercise like a cat the cold water. Surprisingly enough, he seemed to enjoy good health. He also was significantly overweight, a fact the politician considered to be a plus. Touching his ample abdomen, he joked that you should do something good for your body so that your soul could enjoy living in it. When Churchill became Prime Minister of England on May 24, 1940 Dr. Charles McMoran was assigned as his personal physician. He had been the president of the Royal College of Physicians. As Churchill was healthy, initially Dr. McMoran was not very busy. But the good times were over at the end of 1941. Tensions were high because of the Second World War. Pearl Harbor had been bombed by Japanese warplanes. Hitler had declared war against the US. Churchill came for a visit to the US attempting to convince Roosevelt that it would be in the interest of the US to support England in the war against Germany. It was a trying and stressful time, and it had taken its toll on Churchill's health.

On Dec. 27, 1941 Dr. McMoran was called to see Churchill because of chest pains and pains radiating into his left arm. Although Dr. McMoran knew that his patient had hardening of the coronary arteries, he belittled the symptoms and stated that Churchill's blood circulation was a bit sluggish. This was painting a dire situation as a rosy picture. Of course the physician did not want the world to know that the prime Minister was an invalid with a weak heart! This image did not fit into the political arena at that time. Dr. McMoran decided to let the welfare of his country rule over the state of health of his patient, and indeed Churchill was a robust man. He survived this episode, which most likely was a heart attack. Before the war was over Churchill covered 155,000 miles of air travel. It was a grueling schedule, and as a result his health deteriorated: he developed pneumonia when he returned from a conference in Casablanca in January of 1943. He had a chronic cough, likely from congestive heart failure with a superimposed chest infection, but with sulfonamides his pneumonia resolved. Was the problem solved? No, of course it was not; but the image of a strong leader needed to be maintained, and so his busy schedule continued unabated. Following a trip to Teheran and to Cairo he developed another bout of pneumonia. This was at the end of 1943. With reluctance the physician reported to the government in London that Churchill had to "stay in bed for a few days with a cold". A harmless picture was presented and a stiff upper lip maintained. But behind closed doors the situation was not so harmless. Churchill became depressed and had problems breathing because of congestive heart failure. He suffered of the deteriorating blood supply to his ailing heart muscle, but things had to be kept under wraps. Dr. McMoran was assuming the role of the spokesperson for Churchill, and in the doctor's opinion nobody was allowed to learn of Churchill's depression. It would leave a serious dent in the image of this outstanding politician. No, this certainly could not be reported to London! For his honorable efforts Dr. McMoran was knighted in 1942. But even the knighthood of his doctor did not improve Churchill's health. Circulation was not only poor in his heart, but affected his whole body, particularly the circulation to his brain. Churchill started to suffer from memory lapses and Lord McMoran became more and more a kind of general state secretary. Churchill's fighting spirit had faded away, and his political fortunes turned against him at the end of the Second World War. War and destruction were finally over, but the destruction of Churchill's health continued. He suffered a small stroke in August 1949, which caused him to lose his voice - a devastating blow to a previously famous speaker! His depressions became longer and more severe. His spirit however was not broken. Despite all of the difficulties he had to deal with, he was able to rise to power one more time in 1951. His diseased body had other plans, as another stroke in February of 1952 had more debilitating effects. Lord McMoran called this a "certain lability of the brain circulation". This was like labeling a catastrophic atomic blast as a small explosion with minor damages! A further, more severe stroke followed in June 1952, which prevented Churchill temporarily to carry on with his political career. I'm not certain what kind of harmlessly sounding report Dr. McMoran tried to feed to the public at this time, but it was now obvious that Churchill had become a shell of the man who he once was. His party colleagues pressured him to step down in 1955. The downhill course went on in the same fashion: there were more strokes, more depression and more memory loss. But it was only on January 24, 1965 that Churchill finally died at the age of 90. Shortly after his death Lord McMoran felt justified to publish all of the details of his patient's ills in a book, even though he had consistently downplayed Churchill's true state of health before. Churchill was disabled for the last 15 years of his life due to his weak heart and several strokes, which had caused physical impairment, memory loss and depression (Lord McMoran, 2002).

What went wrong with Winston Churchill?

When Winston Churchill entered his career as the Prime Minister in the tumultuous WWII times he was already overweight, if not obese and had cardiovascular risks. With the stress of his job and the endless travels he put an additional burden on his system. He did suffer a heart attack that he survived. Dr. McMoran belittled Churchill's health problems, but eventually his patient did get a series of strokes. This is a disease pattern, which is not unexpected with cardiovascular disease, as the hardening of arteries does not only affect the heart vessels, but also the vessels of the brain. After 15 years of disabilities (memory loss, difficulties moving around) he died at an age of 90. Churchill's health pattern is what obese people have to face. It depends on the genetic make-up whether a person will survive a heart attack or a stroke. In Churchill's case we are looking at a person with a robust constitution, otherwise he would have died much earlier. All the same, robust or not, prevention of his health problems should have started in his 30's or 40's by watching his diet intake through calorie-restriction, doing regular exercise of some kind like walking, sports, dancing etc. and substituting any missing hormones. In Churchill's time very little was known about proper food intake and supplementation with vitamins and minerals. But any physician would have probably raised his hands in despair, as Churchill was no compliant patient! He did not want to participate in any kind of sports, and he loved his cigars. The cigars accelerated the hardening of his arteries and made him more prone to lung infections. The use of bioidentical hormones for prevention of premature aging is only known since the mid 1990's. The goal with regard to Churchill's health would have been to cut down his long period of disability and change this into active years of retirement. But if a patient does not want to give up smoking, does not want to exercise and eats/drinks excessively, there is nothing that can be done to change the outcome. With the patient's deliberate underminingof any well-meaning medical advice even the most brilliant physician could not have made a difference here. For a prominent politician the consequences of a faulty lifestyle apply in the same way as for a person of more humble standing. This is where the "golden years" have seriously derailed. Long lasting disability is not a pleasant way to live to a ripe old age!

Ludwig van Beethoven: damaged by alcohol, finished off by medicine

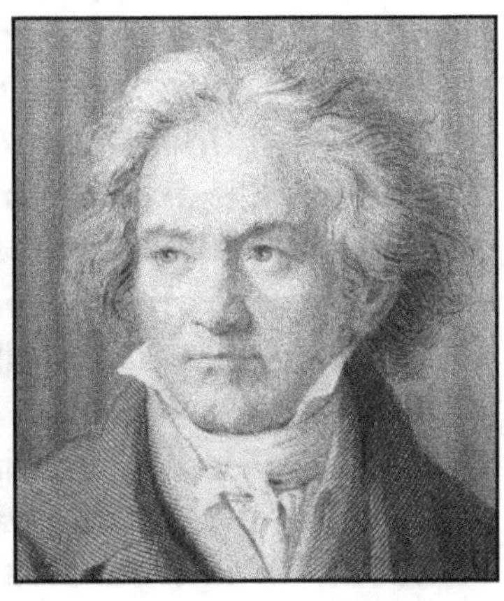

Beethoven along with Mozart is recognized as one of the great Vienna classic composers. Generally people are aware that he lost his hearing early in life, but nevertheless he continued to compose. What is less known is that he had a long history of medical ailments for which he consulted about 10 different physicians throughout his life. None of them could help him.

Beethoven's deafness developed over several years. First there was a history of buzzing and roaring noises in both ears, which started around 1798, when Beethoven was only 28 years old. Dr. Marage brought up the topic of Beethoven's deafness at a conference of the French Academy of Sciences in January 1928 and again in December of 1929. As a result a number of medical experts went over the autopsy report and known medical facts regarding this case and concluded that the famous composer likely had developed a labyrinthitis. It was thought that it might have been triggered by intestinal problems that occurred at the same time. 60% of his hearing had been lost by 1801, and in 1816 at the age of only forty-six Beethoven was completely deaf. Research also turned to several color paintings of the artist. They show a butterfly rash on his cheeks. Several medical experts feel that this could be evidence of lupus, an autoimmune disease. This might also explain some of the abdominal pains as lupus can affect the gastrointestinal system. Lupus can also affect the lining of blood vessels and lead to closure of small

vessels, perhaps of both ears. On the other hand there is a condition, called otosclerosis where one of the hearing bones (the stapes) gets stiff, so sound waves can no longer be transmitted to the inner ear. There is a higher risk of developing otosclerosis in patients who had measles as is explained under references regarding "Beethoven's medical illnesses". Of course in the time before 1800 vaccinations against childhood diseases were unknown, and child mortality was high. Beethoven did have the measles as a small child and small pox a bit later. He also survived typhoid fever. But for a case of otosclerosis there was no help available in the time when the artist suffered from this condition, which was in the early 1800's. Nowadays a relatively small surgical procedure, a stapedectomy, can be performed that would prevent deafness from setting in. But this procedure has only been available since 1956. It is amazing enough that quite a few records are available from such a long time back. Researchers had enough material to study, including an autopsy report that showed excessive skull bone formation, the expected dwindling of the hearing nerves, called nerve atrophy and excessive hardening of the arteries of the inner ear. His brain showed more than average grey matter.

Another important fact is that Beethoven came from an alcoholic family. His father was an alcoholic. Beer and wine were the common drinks, and visiting pubs regularly since the age of 11 was not something that raised many eyebrows in this time. Bottled drinks and juices were not even available at that time and drinking water was highly unsafe, as it was often contaminated. This was also not a time where children and youngsters could drink juice, as keeping foods fresh was nearly impossible. It can be easily assumed that young Ludwig drank beer and wine already as a youngster. Of course this comes with consequences: at one point, sooner or later, the liver function caves in! But there was an additional hazard to drinking wine in the 1800's. Often sour-tasting wines were laced with lead salts to make them more palatable. Nobody gave it any thought that lead could be something harmful. The wine tasted sweeter, and this was all that counted! In the meantime, of course, it is known how toxic lead ingestion is to anybody!

This brings us to the autopsy report again: liver cirrhosis with liver failure was also diagnosed. Associated with this he had what is called portal hypertension, because the cirrhotic liver blocked the blood flow from the gut veins to the liver. The increased pressure in the portal system led to large fluid accumulations in the composer's abdomen medically know as "ascites"). These were drained until before his death and often more than 2 US gallons were removed, which is the equivalent of 8 liters. At the time it was common practice to close the puncture wounds with lead containing soaps. To add to the misery of the composer's last months, he also came down with pneumonia. Dr. Andreas Wawruch, the physician that was consulted, prescribed lead salts to loosen up secretions. This was a customary medication at that time, as antibiotics had not been invented yet. It is not surprising that high amounts of lead were found in Beethoven's hair when the forensic medicine expert Dr. Christian Reiter analyzed it in 2007 on hair probes that had been passed on from generation to generation. He had been thoroughly exposed to lead, starting with wine that was laced with lead salts. Next lead containing soap was used to close wounds, and another insult to the system was the prescription of lead salts to fight pneumonia.

For some time the standard diagnosis of "syphilis" was fashionable among those studying the composer's illnesses. Of course a few wild rumors were in circulation that it was the late effects of syphilis that lead to the severe hearing loss and deafness of the artist. In this case samples of the hair would have been positive for arsenic and mercury. These were the substances in standard treatments used in the 1800's to combat syphilis, but research came up empty. There was no sign of arsenic or mercury in the hair sample, which according to Dr. Reiter excludes the theory that Beethoven's hearing loss would have been from "end stage syphilis". Dr. Reiter concluded that the cause of death was lead poisoning and end stage cirrhosis of the liver.

Beethoven was not an easy patient for his health care providers. If he received a prescription for a medication, he would happily take double of it, thinking that "more is better". Due to his increasing deafness the man was struggling with severe emotional difficulties and also suffered from reoccurring depressions. He was known as a slightly eccentric and tempestuous individual in his younger years, but he became a difficult reclusive and a cantankerous person as time went on. Some experts think Beethoven's regular and sometimes excessive alcohol intake may have triggered the development of a bipolar illness. He was at times suicidal when depressed, but never followed through with any plans. As alcohol had a stimulating effect on Beethoven, one of his physicians, Dr. Johann Malfatti, ordered an alcohol laced ice cream as "medicine" during his last bout of his illness. Beethoven's mood lifted instantly and he responded exclaiming: "Wonder, wonder, wonder...only through Dr. Malfatti's science will I be saved!" He may have felt better for a short while, but unfortunately he was wrong. A few days later, in March of 1827, Beethoven died at the age of only 57 years.

What went wrong with Ludwig van Beethoven?

Unfortunately Beethoven lived at a time when the type of ear surgery that may have saved his hearing had not yet

been invented. The hearing loss of the famous pianist and composer was what drove him to seek the advice of several physicians who ordered various lead containing drugs. The lead containing drugs had severely damaging effects and put him on a destructive path. It was lead poisoning that killed him, and the other avenue to his demise was the end-stage cirrhosis of his liver. Beethoven came from a dysfunctional family where his father was an alcoholic and took him along to pubs when he was only 11 years old. He was exposed to heavy alcohol intake for over 30 years. Even 10 to 15 years of heavy alcohol intake can cause liver cirrhosis. Nowadays his doctor would probably tell him: "Look Ludwig, you have to quit boozing, or next your system is going to quit!" It is doubtful whether the outcome would have been any different. Probably he would have stormed out of the office with a few choice expletives. After all he was a temperamental individual! Beethoven's doctors knew already then that too much alcohol could be a source of health problems, and in his later years he seemed to have been quite moderate with alcohol consumption. By that time however, the damage was already done, and the consequences were painfully obvious: there was the development of portal hypertension that is associated with advanced cirrhosis of the liver. With this condition fluid accumulates in the abdominal cavity and can also lead to pleurisy of the lungs. Often the veins around the lower end of the esophagus become 3 to 4 times the normal size, a condition called esophageal varices. They can burst and lead to death from internal bleeding. He had the fluid accumulations, and he also was poisoned from alcohol sweetened with lead and was further poisoned from the lead contained in the material used to plug the drainage holes from frequent puncture wounds. The physicians had to resort to the punctures as a last-ditch effort to drain the abdominal fluid accumulations. His

relatively short life span and untimely death does not come as a surprise. Patients with end stage liver cirrhosis cannot be expected to live long lives because of complications like liver failure, internal bleeding from esophageal varices and other complications. In his case it was lead poisoning that sent his health on a downhill course, and finally liver cirrhosis with liver failure sealed his fate.

Michael Jackson: This is it; why he died too early

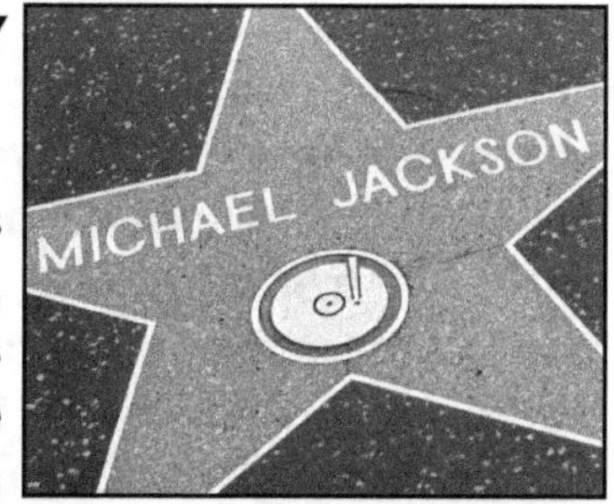

The popular pop singer has been in the public eye for 40 years, first performing with his brothers in the "Jackson 5" from the age of six onwards, later becoming an adult rock star singer and performer. His career suddenly ended 2009 less than three weeks before a planned series of 50 concerts in London, which ironically was entitled "This is it".

While Michael Jackson's career was a steady rise, his health was quite the opposite. Health problems plagued the star already in the mid 1980's. His skin became lighter colored and his facial appearance changed. He was diagnosed with vitiligo and lupus. Vitiligo is an autoimmune disease where the pigment of the skin fades in spots causing a leopard-like appearance. Eventually he had a European complexion when all of his skin had de-pigmented. Michael did not like his appearance and saw many plastic surgeons to improve his features around the nose, the cheeks, the forehead and his lips. He virtually was hooked to plastic surgery! What is worse, the physicians involved probably made not much of an effort to counsel the patient and went along with his demands. Also, to do surgery is more lucrative than not doing surgery... By 1990 he had at least

10 cosmetic surgical procedures on his head. He is thought to have suffered from body dysmorphic disorder, which is a psychological condition where the person is excessively preoccupied with his physical features. The lupus, another autoimmune disease, had affected his face by developing a red rash on his cheeks. It likely also affected the lining of his joints causing. He developed arthritis at an early age. The autopsy report did not mention any organs to be affected by lupus.

Although the press reported that Michael Jackson would have died of a heart attack, the autopsy finding said otherwise. Toxicology tests were ordered, and the results showed that he died of an overdose of the anesthetic Propofol and the anxiety relieving drug lorazepam. Beside those drugs, other medications were found, namely midazolam (Versed), diazepam (Valium), lidocaine and ephedrine. Although the combination of Propofol and lorazepam in high enough doses was enough to suppress the rock star's breathing center, the multiple other drugs in his system (particularly midazolam and diazepam) would have even further suppressed his breathing. Why would the toxicologists find ephedrine? Ephedrine was used in the past for treatment of asthma to open up the bronchial tubes. But in the case of Jackson ephedrine was used as an "upper". This street drug is a derivative of amphetamine, and one of the side effects of ephedrine is insomnia, which would explain the need for sleeping pills as "downers". Some of those, diazepam, lorazepam, or midazolam were also used by Jackson. It is known that the singer suffered from insomnia and he had used sleeping pills in the past. Michael Jackson also used Demerol as far back as 1984 when he had facial burns during the filming of a Pepsi commercial. In the 1990's when he had a broken vertebra from a fall off a stage he used Demerol again. Demerol is highly addictive, and it is thought that he abused this

pain medication on and off. Despite rumors that he would have been killed from an overdose of Demerol, the autopsy report did not support this. In reality it was Propofol in combination with lorazepam, given intravenously by his personal physician, Dr. Conrad Murray. Michael Jackson was only 50 years old.

What went wrong with Michael Jackson?

An intravenous overdose of Propofol and lorazepam is not normally what the doctor orders. But Dr. Conrad Murray took it upon himself to prescribe both medications to his patient Michael Jackson for sleeping or stress relief. It is also known that the artist was pleading with his doctor to give him the strong medications. All he wanted was sleep, and I'm certain that Dr. Murray was also manipulated by the insistence of his patient. It is doubtful whether he had any control over the amount of pills his patient was actually ingesting. The fact remains that he gave him an overdose of medication, which ultimately killed the star. Dr. Murray had some time to think about his therapeutic blunders in jail. In November of 2011 he was found guilty of non-voluntary manslaughter and sentenced to four years in jail. Due to overcrowding in the institution and the fact that he was showing good behavior he got out after two years. Lucky for him!

So far we have seen just the end point of a life that was cut short due to medical mismanagement. However, the problems started already in Michael Jackson's childhood when his father physically abused him. In other words, he came from a dysfunctional family, and the trauma he had to endure as a child had an utterly negative impact on his mental and physical well being later in his life. His body dysmorphic disorder likely was related to this as well. Other psychiatric conditions (anxiety, chronic insomnia, mood disorders) are often also associated with having

been brought up in a toxic family setting. Next he was under the pressure of being in the limelights as a childhood star. It is questionable whether there was love and affection to allow him to thrive, but it is certain that there were plenty of high, if not unreasonable expectations. Michael Jackson was set on the pathway of pain and anxiety early. He took medications like any patient who is desperate to feel better, but there is no medication for emotional pain. The exposure to powerful narcotics, pain pills and anti-anxiety drugs would also have their consequences, one of them being personality changes. In a world of make-belief, glaring lights, reporters, applause and glamor the human touch must have been painfully absent. More than drugs the singer and performer would have needed a compassionate psychologist who would have counseled him over the course of several years. Cognitive therapy and clinical hypnotherapy could have been used to reprogram the bad memories engrained into Michael's subconscious from childhood on and to help the patient to get rid of any repressed anger. Some studies show that autoimmune diseases develop in individuals who have repressed anger; it is the response of the immune system that turns against the body. In this sense vitiligo and lupus likely were the tip of an iceberg as outward signs of a deeper psychological problem in the life of Michael Jackson.

The entire course of events is an example that drugs cannot solve emotional problems. Taken in moderation they can diminish anxiety and can be used as a temporary means to treat depression. But each drug has its own side-effect profile, which needs to be carefully balanced against the benefits. Less is more! Without the overdose of Propofol and lorazepam Michael Jackson would still be with us.

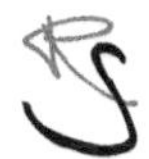

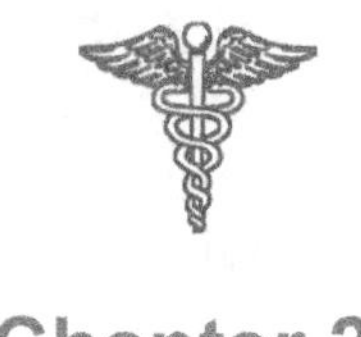

Chapter 2:

How Modern Drugs Come and Go

The physician's desk reference is published once per year. It lists all of the side effects of prescription drugs and is handed out to any practicing physician. Computer programs are also available that help the treating physician to recognize possible drug interactions when multiple drugs are used to treat several ailments in the same patient. The drug industry attempts to work together with physicians to communicate adverse reactions to the health profession; physicians in turn report any adverse reactions they have noted regarding prescription drugs back to the drug industry. And everybody who has ever received some prescription medication may remember that he also received a printed note from the pharmacist. It listed all the likely and even the less likely side effects of the prescription. It almost sounds like a warning: use at your own risk!

There are medications that initially received the blessings of the FDA, but some time later they are axed. I cite one example, a medication for arthritis under the name

of VIOXX. While it was first considered as innocuous, a sudden voluntary withdrawal showed the dark side of the drug. The medication was initially developed as an anti-arthritis drug, which had fewer side effects on the stomach than the older naproxen drug, leading to less bleeding ulcers. But as time went on evidence of VIOXX related side effects were mounting, such as heart attacks and strokes. The company Merck withdrew the drug voluntarily. This was a temporary setback to the drug industry. It was confusing: why would a more specific medicine with less side effects in one area (less ulcers) suddenly have side effects in another area (heart attacks and strokes)?

The answer may come from another similar fiasco, namely from the Women's Health Initiative in 2002. This was a clinical trial involving over 16,000 postmenopausal women. It has taught physicians a tough lesson: you cannot mess with nature's hormone receptors or else you create a risk of strokes (41%), heart attacks (29%), blood clots (twice as many), breast cancer (26%), colorectal cancer (37%) and you increase Alzheimer's disease (by 76%). In these trials women were given Premarin, which are horse-derived estrogens and Provera, which is a synthetic progesterone-like molecule instead of a bio-identical hormone. These horse estrogens and synthetic hormones do not fit to the natural estrogen and progesterone receptors in a woman's body, but function like "xenohormones", which have a remote estrogenic effect. The end result was that physicians inadvertently created estrogen dominance in these women, which unbalanced the whole endocrine system of the treated women causing the above-mentioned complications. If the treating physicians had put postmenopausal women on bio-identical hormones (bio-identical estrogen and bio-identical progesterone) these women would simply have felt younger for longer without any nefarious side effects. But this was not the objective of the study! The

objective had been to prove that Premarine and Provera would be good for the cardiovascular system and prevent osteoporosis. It is most unfortunate for those who were treated with synthetic hormones that they paid with their health or even with their lives for this type of research. For Big Pharma it meant that they would not be able to make a booming business from the increased sales of synthetic hormones. For people, the consumers it reinforced the warning: buyer beware!

Synthetic hormones like Premarine and Provera have a list of side effect that are hazardous to women's health. HDL cholesterol gets diminished and LDL cholesterol gets elevated causing the heart attack and stroke risk. With bioidentical hormones the opposite is true: HDL cholesterol gets elevated and LDL cholesterol is reduced, which effectively postpones hardening of the arteries preventing heart attacks and strokes. Through their reproductive years women gain a 10-year survival advantage over men from the regular estrogen production of their ovaries, balanced by the cyclical progesterone production. Anti-aging physicians have prescribed bio-identical hormones safely to postmenopausal women without any side effects. They say that bio-identical hormones can be given life-long and women's lives can be prolonged a total of 15 to 20 years by giving bio-identical estrogen along with bio-identical progesterone starting immediately after menopause. Incidentally the same is true for men when they get into the change of life (male menopause or andropause) where testosterone levels decline. Simply adding back bioidentical testosterone will prolong men's lives as well.

Many physicians still deny the results of the Women's Health Initiative and they continue to prescribe the same synthetic hormones, just at lower doses and for a shorter period of time (up to five years) hoping that this would lead to less side-effects. Common sense should indicate that what is a poison at a higher dose is still a poison at a lower dose, even when given for a shorter period of time. And what is the physician to do after the 5 years have passed? Abandon the patient?

Not everything is bad about Big Pharma. There have been very encouraging developments by the drug industry in the past with regard to asthma treatments and blood pressure medications. Before the newer receptor-specific medications were developed, asthma was treated with ephedrine. This is a medication, which stimulates both beta-1 and beta-2 receptors. Beta-1 receptors are found in the heart muscle leading to heart muscle contractions, beta-2 receptors are found in smooth muscles such as the bronchial tubes. Ephedrine stimulated both of these receptors. As ephedrine is an amphetamine derivative, there is potential for addiction to develop. So ephedrine was a lousy drug for an asthmatic, because it was not specific for the bronchial tubes. It had serious side effects on the heart and could cause heart attacks and sudden death from heart arrhythmias in elderly patients. Fortunately salbutamol was invented in 1968 and marketed as the Ventolin inhaler for asthmatics. This is a selective beta-2 activator (physicians call it “beta-2 receptor agonist”). While asthma is still a difficult condition, treating it has become much safer. Thoroughly researched and safe medications are helping many patients to live full and productive normal lives.

With regard to treatment of the heart and the arteries, the beta-blockers have been developed. The first such drug was propranolol (Inderal), which had been developed by James W. Black in the 1960’s. He was awarded the Nobel Prize in medicine for its discovery in 1988. Inderal slows down the heartbeat, lowers blood pressure and helps alleviate chest pains from coronary artery spasms (angina pains). Propranolol is a non-specific beta-1 and beta-2 receptor blocker. Because of the beta-2 blocking activity asthmatics cannot take it, as it would make their asthma worse.

The detection of all kinds of receptors distributed in the body tissues has stimulated the drug industry to develop new more specific medications with the promise of fewer side effects.

Developing new drugs can be complicated and often takes several years. After biochemical tests are completed the new drug is tested on animals to establish the effects of the drug and test for toxic side effects. If the drug is a hopeful candidate for humans, it undergoes a 3-phase trial with phase 3 being the last rigid test (See link under references that explains this regarding an example of Alzheimer drug development). The regulatory bodies throughout the world, in the US it is the FDA, will now review the data and either approve of it or reject it.

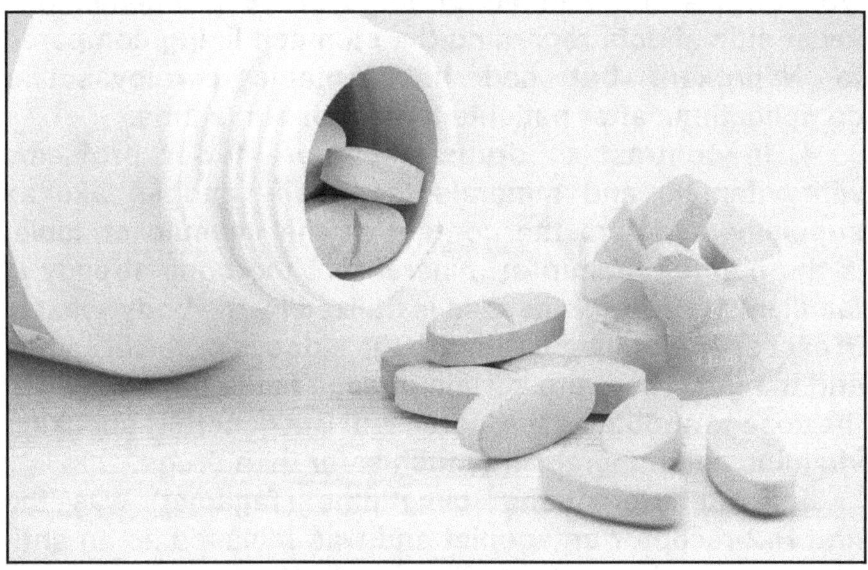

There are problems with this approach:

1. The new drug has to be able to be patented or it will not pay for the drug company to go through the expensive

drug development process. Many natural substances with less side effects are not manufactured, because it would not be profitable to do so.

2. As seen with the Women's Health Initiative, the modification of the hormone molecules made it impossible for the woman's body to recognize the synthetic hormone and multiple life threatening complications set in instead. Despite greed (drug company) and regulations (FDA) synthetic hormones will not fit the body receptors the way nature does it on its own with the natural hormones. A hormon substance will always be a substitute prone to causing side effects unless it is the body's bio-identical hormone.

3. Unexpected side effects can occur even years after the safe release of a drug as seen with VIOXX. It was a wonderful anti-inflammatory for arthritic problems, had lower side effects regarding the stomach lining compared to Naproxen, but had unacceptable cardiovascular complications after patients took it for some time.

4. In contrast to drugs, there are fewer problems with vitamins and minerals that many people take as supplements. Here the content of the capsule or tablet is the natural vitamin or mineral that the body already is familiar with. What is needed is utilized by the body, what is in excess is eliminated through the kidneys or the liver, bile and the gut. There are certain dosage limits beyond which the dosage should not be increased! But generally speaking vitamins and minerals are much safer than drugs.

5. Drug interactions: cimetidine (Tagamet) was the first H-2-receptor antagonist and was released as an anti-ulcer medication in 1979. This medication has practically eliminated the need for surgery for most duodenal ulcers. However, years after release of this important medication it became apparent that an important detoxification enzyme system in liver cells called cytochrome P450 or CYP3A4

is inhibited by Cimetidine. The same detoxification system in the liver also detoxifies erythromycin and there are a host of drugs that are eliminated in the same way such as antidepressants. This leads to an elevation of the blood levels of both drugs when a patient on cimetidine takes erythromycin for an infection. A brief overview of the myriad of drugs that are eliminated via the cytochrome P 450 enzyme detoxification system in the liver is listed under references. The more medication you take, the more likely it will be that the physician has to make adjustments regarding safe doses. To complicate matters, people can be fast and slow metabolizers due to genetic variances with regard to how the liver metabolizes drugs and this has become an important factor when prescribing antidepressants.

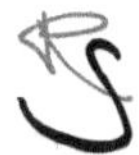

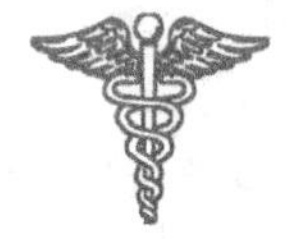

Chapter 3:

Treating Symptoms Rather Than the Cause

Generally patients do not come to the doctor's office to get just preventative tests, like "doctor, I need to get checked, just to be sure that everything is well." Usually there are symptoms that bring patients to the doctor's office. A hacking cough can be the symptom. But further investigation by the doctor is necessary to establish the cause. Is the diagnosis a bad cold, asthma, or another form of disease? It is the diagnosis that determines what treatment will be required. Treating only symptoms leads to poor medicine. Let us look for instance at one buzzword called "erectile dysfunction". It is a symptom, not a diagnosis. It simply means a man has a problem with erections. But the ads from the drug industry have conditioned people to think that Viagra, Cialis or other such drugs would be required to overcome this problem: one little blue pill can do it. It's shown on TV commercials that everybody is happy! This is jumping to conclusions. Good medicine asks the doctor to do a thorough history on his patient: did the man have normal erections in the past or not?

Are there concomitant illnesses like high blood pressure, cardiovascular disease, diabetes etc. present? Could it be that the patient is testosterone hormone deficient? In the case of a hypertensive that is on diuretic medication a simple switch to an alternative medication may restore his previously normal erections. In a testosterone deficient male bioidentical testosterone hormone replacement will normalize the situation. So, it is important to look for the cause of the patient's symptoms, perhaps do some clarifying tests and then treat the cause, not the symptom. This may not be a case for the little blue pill!

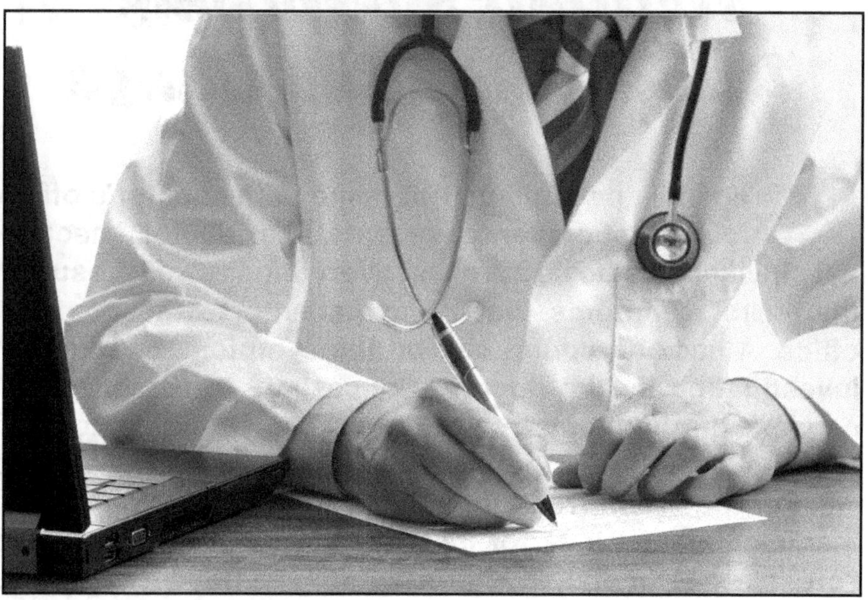

The average patient today

After reading the first chapter earlier, you may say that most of these celebrities lived a long time ago and their stories do not relate to you and me. But they still do! The following example shows that prescriptions can be a potential minefield for patients. Instead of getting better they get into the muddle of side effects.

Here is an example of Joe, the mechanic down the street who is about 40 years old. He simply does not feel well and has noticed a lack of energy lately. His wife sent him to the doctor for a complete physical. The doctor found that the patient's blood pressure was moderately elevated. He sent him for some blood work as well and during the repeat visit the blood pressure is still high. The blood tests revealed an elevated cholesterol level. So the doctor prescribes a water pill (diuretic) for the high blood pressure and atorvastatin (Lipidil) to lower Joe's cholesterol. On the next visit Joe's blood pressure has normalized. The patient feels more energetic, but now he has a cold. When the doctor listens to Joe's lungs, he is concerned as the lung sounds are abnormal. The doctor thinks that Joe is suffering from a bad bronchitis. As the patient is allergic to penicillin, the antibiotic erythromycin is prescribed instead. After only a few days Joe develops extreme muscle pains and sees the doctor again. At that point the doctor realizes that there was an interaction between erythromycin and Lipidil. Both of the drugs are deactivated in the liver by the cytochrome P450 pathway leading to higher than normal levels when both drugs are combined. This accounts for the problems of the patient. Erythromycin is discontinued as the patient's lungs are now clear. Fortunately for Joe all of the muscle pains dissolve without permanent damage. In the literature though a condition is described, called rhabdomyolysis where permanent muscle damage can lead to the acute release of myoglobin from dying muscle tissue that is released into the blood. This can clog up the kidneys, which in turn can cause acute renal failure. There are cases known where the patient ended up with permanent dialysis as a result of drug interaction (toxicity through the cytochrome P450 pathway). Luckily Joe did not get any of that! But let me continue with the story of Joe.

When Joe reported his muscle aches to the physician, he also mentioned that lately he was experiencing erectile dysfunction. He wondered whether Cialis would not help that problem, because he has seen a TV commercial about this recently. The doctor explained to Joe that developing erectile dysfunction at the age of 40 would be unusual; he would be too young for that. Nevertheless, he did prescribe Cialis for Joe to keep him happy. About 1 month later Joe reports to the doctor that Cialis worked just fine, but he had developed chest pains and migraine headaches. The doctor measured Joe's blood pressure and noticed that it was too high-again. He asked whether the patient still took the water pill. Joe answered that he did. The doctor was worried that Joe may have developed a heart attack and called an ambulance to sent Joe to the hospital. A cardiologist saw him right away. He felt that Cialis had given Joe the side effects of migraines, chest pains (angina) and the elevated blood pressure. Cialis is actually contraindicated (meaning it should not be taken) for patients with high blood pressure. The water pill was also discontinued, as the cardiologist thought it was responsible for the erectile dysfunction. He put Joe on losartan (Cozaar) to lower his blood pressure. The cardiologist also noticed that Joe had gained about 50 pounds of weight in the past 2 years. He explained to Joe and his wife that the weight gain likely was what had caused the high blood pressure and high cholesterol in the first place. Within one week the family doctor measured Joe's blood pressure again, and it was normal. Joe's erections had also returned spontaneously as losartan does not have the side effect that the diuretic has. All the other side effects were gone. The cardiologist had written a summary of his consultation with Joe and his wife at the hospital and sent a copy to the family doctor; he had suggested that the family doctor should follow up with regard to lifestyle factors as there would be a good

possibility that Joe may get off the medications altogether, if he became physically more active and lost a significant amount of weight. Joe liked the idea of perhaps being able to get off the medication. His wife suggested that they adopt a dog from a shelter and go for regular long walks. They did this and they also watched their calorie intake by switching to less processed foods and more vegetables. Within the course of 2 years Joe was able to shed 55 pounds. His body mass index had normalized and he was able to reduce and eventually stop both losartan and atorvastatin. His blood pressure was back to normal and the cholesterol values were normal as well.

Part of the story sounds like a medical nightmare. The patient gets a medication, and at the heels of taking a prescription a few nasty side effects develop! It sounds better, when appropriate medications can limit side effects, but the real winner is a change of lifestyle that enables the patient to enjoy good health. This is a story with a happy ending. But we also know that not all stories come to a good end.

Comments: **This is an example what kind of problems can develop in the health care system with a patient who has high cholesterol levels and high blood pressure. The drug interaction between the antibiotic erythromycin and the cholesterol lowering agent losartan almost damaged Joe's muscles and kidneys permanently (rhabdomyolysis). Joe's side-effect to the diuretic (erectile dysfunction) and his experience with the treatment using Cialis is another example of how dangerous it can be to just treat a symptom. Joe could have developed a full-blown heart attack or a stroke as a side effect of Cialis, because he was a high-risk patient for these complications. The cardiologist was very helpful in sorting out Joe's medications leaving out the ones that caused him trouble. By concentrating on the**

cause of high cholesterol and high blood pressure, namely lifestyle issues (faulty diet and lack of exercise leading to metabolic syndrome) Joe was able to solve his medical problem without medication. It takes a lot of motivation and willpower to follow through on lifestyle changes, but Joe was able to do it with the help of his wife.

Summary about "Treating symptoms rather than the cause"

Many doctors hear of a patient's symptoms and start treating these with various medicines rather than thinking of what the underlying cause of their patient's symptoms is. We have seen this with the celebrities discussed earlier, but we also learnt that this is still the case today (as Joe's example showed). The confusing part in medicine is the fact that we do not know all of the causes for all of the diseases. Often physicians are at a loss to find the reason for diseases like cancer, MS, autoimmune diseases and other problems.

But we do know a lot of causes for many illnesses. Hundred years ago smoking was not looked at as a health hazard, and nobody would have even given a second thought to the hazard of secondary smoke. In the meantime we are fully aware that cigarette smoking causes lung cancer and causes cardiovascular disease. It also causes a number of other cancers. Quitting to smoke, or even better never to smoke, makes a lot of sense in terms of preventing disease.

In the past Twinkies, Dingdongs and Donuts did not quite have the bad name they have in human nutrition as today. But, like with cigarette smoking, we know a bit more what fat, sugar and starch in our food will do to our bodies. First high lipid levels are caused by too much sugar and starch. This in turn causes fat deposits in the arteries, which later calcify and cause arteriosclerosis (narrowing

of the arteries). The ultimate result is death from heart attacks and strokes. It makes a lot of sense to cut back on sugar, fat and starchy food intake and to supplement your diet with high doses of omega-3 fatty acids (molecularly distilled to remove mercury impurities).

In the past the most well known hormones were thyroid hormone and insulin. In the meantime we also know a lot more about hormone changes due to aging. As we will discuss later in more detail, when we age (women above 35, men above 55), there are significant hormonal changes that take place. We can just treat the symptoms associated with this and miss the underlying cause of hormone deficiency. Or we can face the fact of hormone deficiency, have tests to establish what hormones are missing and replace what's missing with bioidentical hormones. This powerful tool can add 15 to 20 years to your life without disabilities when started early enough.

Whenever you experience symptoms, ask yourself first what the cause may be before you rush into taking any medicine. Often simple lifestyle changes can make a significant difference!

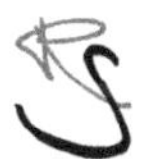

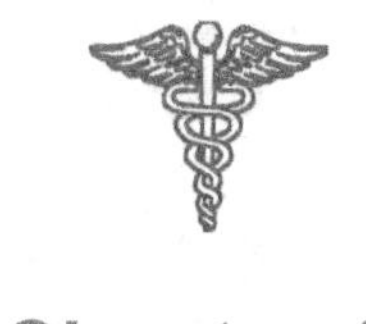

Chapter 4:

Preventing Illness, Concept of Anti-Aging

The thought of preventing illness is not new. But since the mid 1990's it seems that the momentum regarding disease prevention has reached a new level of awareness among the public. The "Prevention" magazine, the "Life extension" magazine, Suzanne Somers' books and the A4M (American Academy of Anti-Aging Medicine) have all helped to re-educate the public about the importance of prevention in health care. Some universities like Harvard University and the Loyola University seem to have embraced this concept as well. Others including many physicians and specialists are somewhat slower in adapting to the new changes.

Here I would like to discuss some of the concepts of anti-aging. With "anti-aging" is meant a delay of aging, not "eternal living". There is a lot of scientific evidence that can explain why prevention is more powerful than attempting to cure a disease later.

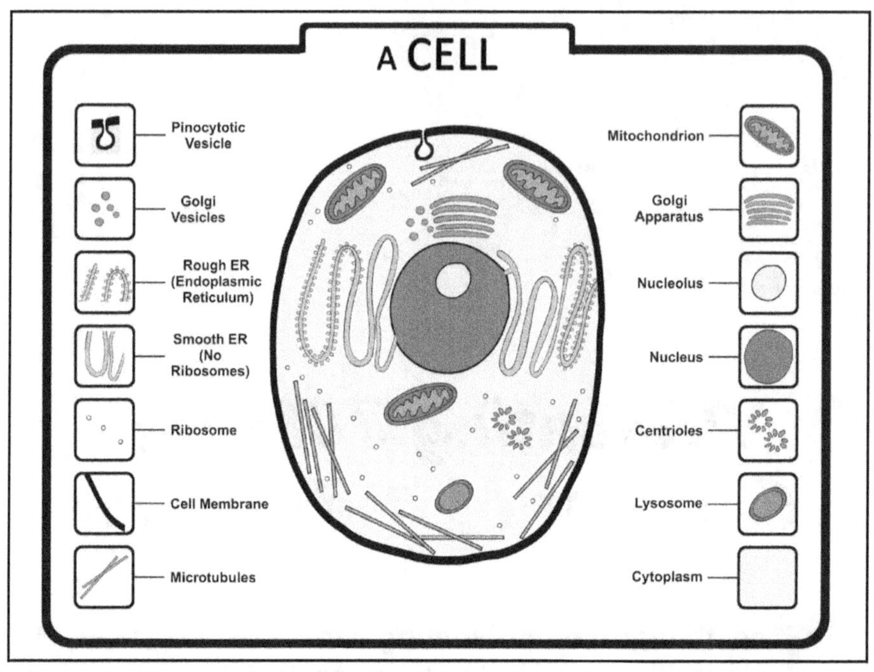

Mitochondria, the energy packages of the cell

At the center of energy production is the mitochondrion, which is a small sub-part of the cell, called an organelle. Each cell has many mitochondria and heart cells have thousands of mitochondria within it. The biochemical citric acid cycle, also called Krebs cycle, is located within the mitochondria. This is where ATP (abbreviation for "adenosine triphosphate") is produced as an energy storing substance. It functions like a living battery that stores energy chemically and releases it again when it is needed. We all know that without energy we could not live. We inherit the mitochondria in our body cells from our mother. The egg contains mitochondria, but the sperm from our father left the mitochondria behind in the tail of the sperm that is not absorbed by the fertilized egg.

There is good evidence that the function of our mitochondria can deteriorate over time with exposure to toxic substances, like pesticides, mercury, pollutants etc. The aging process itself can cause mitochondria to function at a lower level of performance. Fibromyalgia is one of the conditions where mitochondrial function is impaired. Patients with fibromyalgia complain about a chronic lack of energy.

On the other hand, the anti-aging branch of medicine (represented by the American Academy of Anti-Aging Medicine) has provided evidence that the body can be cleansed with chelation treatments utilizing intravenous vitamin C and EDTA or glutathione to flush out toxic materials, especially heavy metals. These antioxidants free the mitochondria from the burdens of accumulated toxins and restore the biochemistry pathways that provide the body with energy. There are also mutations that can occur in mitochondria and they differ between various tissues. Mitochondria of muscle tissue do not have as many mitochondrial mutations as mitochondria of kidney or heart cells. This means that different tissues of the body may age at different rates. It is this area of genetic differences among people that may explain why certain families have a longevity trait, while others don't. It is thought that free radicals, which are highly aggressive toxic metabolic byproducts, can lead to mutations of the DNA of cells and of the DNA of mitochondria. The key of the anti-aging approach is to attempt to minimize the damage by free radicals to cells and mitochondria thus prolonging the span of normal body function.

The mitochondrial concentrations per cell vary from a few mitochondria per cell in metabolically less active tissues versus several thousand mitochondria per cell in metabolically active tissues like the heart, liver, kidneys or skeletal muscles. The weakest organ that develops a

malfunction will determine when the downhill spiral begins, which eventually can lead to death. Typically one of the limiting key organs that can trigger this process can be the heart, the brain, the kidneys, the liver, the lungs, the gut or the bone marrow.

In this context it is useful to know that vitamins and supplements can support the body's metabolism including the mitochondria.

In chapter 12 we will come back to a much more detailed discussion about anti-aging. However, I wanted to prepare you that when the energy metabolism of the mitochondria powerhouses is damaged by free radicals, this could be a cause for developing cancer in any organ.

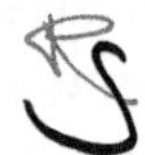

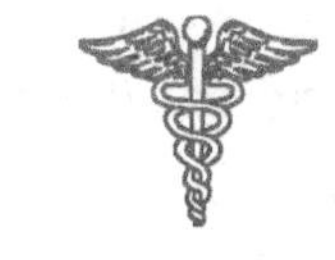

Chapter 5:

Keep a Healthy Brain

Our brain is where all our knowledge is preserved, where our feelings are located, where we think, experience, and define who we are. When everything is working well, we tend to forget about our brain. But when dementia and Alzheimer's sets in, everything changes. In the following section emphasis is placed on preventing this from happening. I will deal with how to preserve your memory step by step. An explanatory section about brain atrophy and how to avoid it follows. As alcohol robs you of memory, you will find a description about alcohol and its effects on your health and on your brain.

Preserve your memory

At the 22nd Annual A4M Las Vegas Conference in mid December 2014 Pamela Smith gave a presentation named "How To Maintain Memory At Any Age". She gave a comprehensive overview of what you can do to prevent Alzheimer's disease. The better we understand the causes of Alzheimer's the more we can interfere with the biochemical processes that lead to Alzheimer's or dementia. Various parts of the brain have different functions like pattern recognition, interpreting auditory and visual stimuli and so on. In the past it was thought that once the brain is developed, it would be stationary until we die. Brain researchers have shown a different picture: the brain continues to develop even after the teenage years. New brain cells can develop as long as we live and new synapses, the connections between brain cells can form all the time. This is called neuroplasticity.

There are detrimental influences like lack of sleep. It causes insulin levels to rise, which in turn causes a lack of memory. Alzheimer's disease has been termed diabetes type 3 because of this close connection of memory loss and uncontrolled high blood sugar levels. In fact diabetics are three times more likely to develop Alzheimer's disease.

There are several subunits of the brain like the hypothalamus, thalamus, hippocampus and the amygdalae, which are important for normal brain function and memory. The hippocampus in particular is a major memory-processing unit, which indexes, constructs and rearranges memories.

Apart from the anatomy of the brain, neurotransmitters are important for the proper functioning of the various parts. Although there are more than 100 of them the most important neurotransmitters are acetylcholine, GABA, glutamate, dopamine and serotonin. Each of these neurotransmitters binds to only one specific receptor before a signal can be sent from one neuron to the next. There is a decline in the speed of neurotransmission with age and also a memory decline. Compared to the memory in a young person a person at the age of 75 has a decline in memory function of about 40%.

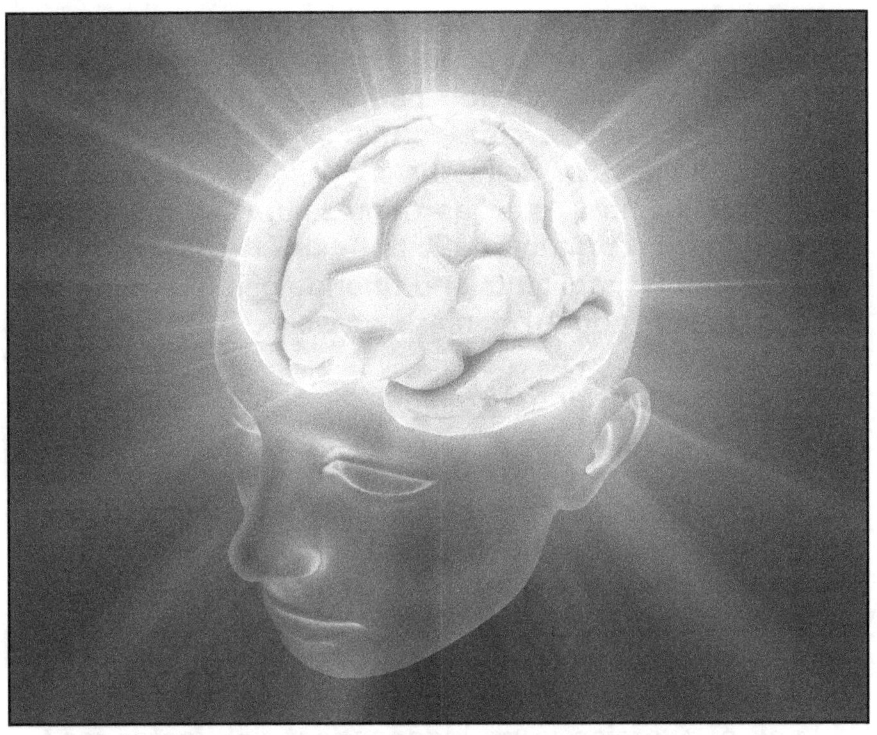

Why do people experience memory decline?

Apart from genetic predisposition the majority of people come down with Alzheimer's disease due to neglecting the body and their brain. Neglecting elevated blood pressure by not treating it properly with medication will lead to vascular dementia. As already mentioned earlier hyperinsulinemia (too much insulin in the blood) from obesity, untreated type 2 diabetes and metabolic syndrome are other factors that predispose a person to Alzheimer's. Lack of exercise is associated with a higher risk of developing Alzheimer's, so is insomnia and a lack of sleep (less than 7 hours per night). With aging there is often poor nutrition, lack of absorption of nutrients, inflammatory bowel conditions

with poor absorption of nutrients and body inflammation. A significant portion of the population is deficient for various enzymes in the methylation pathway, which can lead to high homocysteine levels, the danger of premature heart attacks and vascular dementia. Psychological health can also affect memory loss, as depression and anxiety are associated with cognitive deficits. Toxins like heavy metals, fuels, pesticides, solvents and fluoride can over time lead to memory loss and Alzheimer's as well.

Lifestyle habits and Alzheimer's

There are many lifestyles that cause memory loss: too much stress (from high cortisol levels that damage the hippocampus); smoking that damages acetylcholine receptors; chronic alcohol abuse leads to memory problems from the toxic effect of alcohol on brain cells, which in turn causes a unbalance of serotonin, endorphins and acetylcholine in the hippocampus.

Lack of exercise is an independent risk factor for the development of Alzheimer's disease. Exercise increases the blood supply of the brain, strengthens neural connections and leads to growth of neurons, the basic building blocks of the brain. Mood-regulating neurotransmitters are increased by exercise (serotonin, endorphins).

Sleep deprivation leads to memory loss, but so does the use of aspartame, the artificial sweetener of diet sodas.
Too many refined carbs which get metabolized within 30 minutes into sugar cause oxidization of LDL cholesterol and plaque formation of all the blood vessels including the ones going to the brain and to the heart. Sugar consumption will be as devastating: it hits the system like a bomb! On the long-term this slows down the memory, and you call it "forgetfulness". Once the nutrient flow and the oxygen flow are severely impaired, things come to a grinding halt, and you call the condition dementia or Alzheimer's.

Hormone changes

A lack of testosterone in men and a lack of estrogen in women interferes with cognition and memory. For this reason it is important after menopause and andropause (=the male menopause) to replace missing hormones with the help of a knowledgeable health professional.

Too much DHEA from stress can decrease memory, but too little DHEA from aging can also do this. Alzheimer's patients have DHEA levels that are 48% lower than men and women of the same age who have normal memories. Pregnenolone is a precursor of DHEA, estrogen, progesterone and testosterone. Dr. Smith called pregnenolone the "hormone of memory in the body". At an age of 75 most people have a 65% lower level of pregnenolone than persons in the mid 30's. Pregnenolone keeps your brain balanced between excitation and inhibition, helps you to cope with stress and gives you energy. But before you consider supplementing with pregnenolone, hormone levels should be ordered by a knowledgeable health professional. Just getting a supplement and popping a pill can be compared to lighting a fire with a dynamite stick. Things can get out of control, as dosing can be tricky. Too much pregnenolone can result in too much DHEA, estrogen, progesterone or testosterone. So, don't do this on your own!

Progesterone is manufactured inside the brain, spinal cord and nerves from its precursor, pregnenolone, but in women it also comes from the ovaries until the point of menopause. Progesterone is needed in the production of the myelin sheaths of nerves and it has a neuroprotective function. In menopausal women bioidentical progesterone replacement is a part of Alzheimer's prevention.

Melatonin is a hormone, a powerful antioxidant and a neurotransmitter at the same time. It helps in the initiation of sleep, stimulates the immune system and protects from the toxic effects of cobalt, which has been found to be high in Alzheimer's patients.

Other factors contributing to Alzheimer's

Any inflammatory condition can trigger destruction of neurons, so do the beta-amyloid proteins associated with Alzheimer's. Contributory factors can be food allergies, unbalance of gut bacteria, recreational drugs (particularly ecstasy) and certain medications. Dr. Smith stated that the most common foods causing allergies that affect the brain are: sugar, wheat, dairy, eggs, shellfish, potatoes, beef, tomatoes, corn, coffee, peanuts, roasted soy beans and yeast. To go about it scientifically, there are food sensitivity tests available that give you information on about two hundred common foods and whether you are sensitive to some of them.

Dr. Smith mentioned that the following medications can affect memory: statins, sedatives, steroids, levodopa, muscle relaxants; antihypertensive drugs, antidepressants, antibiotics, anticonvulsants, anti-arrhythmic drugs, pain relieving drugs (analgesics) and antihistamines. If you are on any of these, you may want to discuss alternatives with your doctor. Dr. Perlmutter mentioned that statins interfere with brain function and that they can lead to Alzheimer's.

Promoting brain health

Medication helps only to stall further memory loss for up to 6 months, so Dr. Smith's comment about medications was only this: "much research is still needed in this area".

On the other hand she stated that many foods, vitamins and supplements in combination could improve memory and prevent the development of Alzheimer's disease. She spent considerable time in the remainder of her talk on details regarding foods, vitamins and supplements.

Dr. Smith emphasized the importance of eating foods that are rich in antioxidants like blueberries, apples, raspberries, blackberries and strawberries; cherries, cranberries, cooked kale, garlic, grapes, prunes, raisins and raw spinach. But at the same time she stressed that we cannot trust the food industry anymore, and we need to buy organic foods. She gave an example of the "dirty dozen" as defined by the environmental working group.

Food intake also applies to portions: eat 5 to 6 smaller meals per day. Consume red meat at the most three times per week. Less is better! Other authors say that once or twice per week is the limit for grass fed beef.

The brain needs fats like nuts and seeds: walnuts, almonds, pine nuts etc.

Fish also contains healthy omega-3 fatty acids and DHA. The problem with predator fish like tuna or swordfish is their contamination with mercury. But wild salmon and mackerel are still OK. A good alternative is supplementation with pharmaceutical grade EPA/DHA omega-3 capsules. They are molecularly distilled, which means they are not contaminated with mercury or PBC's and they are more concentrated; they typically contain 1000 to 1400 mg of EPA/DHA per capsule (available at health food stores). One to two capsules twice per day (a total of 2 to 4 per day) would be a good anti-inflammatory dose. People with arthritis may want to supplement with 3 capsules twice per day to control the inflammation.

Specific food recommendations

Use olive oil and coconut oil for cooking; avoid the omega-6 oils (safflower oil, grape seed oil, sunflower oil, corn oil to just mention a few). These latter oils, which are heavily advertised by the food industry, create too much

arachidonic acid leading to body inflammation. Your brain is very sensitive to inflammation, which causes Alzheimer's. For the same reason avoid deep fried foods and processed foods.

There is more you need to watch for: no food additives, no artificial food colorings, no preservatives, flavors and MSG. Be alert about the food industry's alternative "language" or terminology for MSG: "natural flavor", "yeast extract" etc.

Brain nutrients

Dr. Smith reviewed a long list of brain nutrients that support the brain in its metabolism and prevent the development of dementia and Alzheimer's disease.

I will only highlight the most effective and established nutrients here.

DHA: It has been known since 1999 that Alzheimer's patients are missing DHA in their system. Molecularly distilled fish oil with high omega-3 fatty acids (both EPA and DHA) is one of the mainstays of prevention of inflammation in the body and the brain. 2 capsules twice per day of the concentrated 1000mg to 1400 mg capsules are desirable to prevent Alzheimer's disease.

Phosphatylserine (PS): This phospholipid is part of the membrane of brain cells and controls what nutrients enter into them. It also increases the neurotransmitters acetylcholine, serotonin, norepinephrine, epinephrine and dopamine. Dr. Smith mentioned that PS is naturally present in foods like brown rice, fish, soy and green vegetables (particularly the leafy ones). The daily dosage recommended by Dr. Smith is 300 mg (note: some people develop a bothersome, but harmless bitter taste in the mouth at this dose; in this case take a lower dose like 100 or 200 mg per day).

Ginkgo Biloba: It improves blood flow to the brain and counteracts shrinkage of the hippocampus with age. Dr. Smith recommends 60 mg to 240 mg daily.

Alpha Lipoic Acid: Alpha lipoic acid is an antioxidant; it helps stimulating the sprouting of new nerve cells and nerve fibers. Take 100 mg of alpha lipoic acid daily for memory.

Dr. Smith recommended many other supplements, which I will not explain in detail here: B vitamins, vitamin E and C, carnosine, acetyl-L-carnitine, boron, ginger, coenzyme Q-10 (or CoQ-10), curcumin, vinpocetine, zinc, grape seed extract, blueberry extract, Ashwaganda, glyceryl-phosphoryl-choline, same, huperzine A and DMAE.

When the benefits of taking CoQ-10 were discussed, Dr. Smith reminded the audience "whatever is good for the heart, is good for the brain". She recommended reading Dr. Perlmutter's book from which this phrase was borrowed.

Genetic factors

Dr. Smith pointed out that there are about 5 genes that have been detected which are associated with Alzheimer's disease and in addition the apolipoprotein E4 (APOE4). About 30% of people carry this gene, yet only about 10% get Alzheimer's disease, which shows how important lifestyle factors are (in medical circles this is called epigenetic factors) to suppress the effect of the APOE4 gene. She also stated that our genes contribute only about 20% to the overall risk of developing Alzheimer's disease. This leaves us with 80% of Alzheimer's cases where we can use the brain nutrients discussed above coupled with regular exercise to improve brain function.

Conclusion

Don't wait for a magic pill to be developed by Big Pharma. Follow the simple steps in combination that Dr. Pamela Smith talked about in her presentation:

- exercise
- have organic food to keep toxins out of your body and brain
- replace missing hormones with bioidentical ones
- take supplements that are known to be effective

In other words provide the right environment for your genes to work properly without getting Alzheimer's disease.

Avoid brain atrophy

When the 24-year old football player Chris Borland suddenly decides to quit his active sports career, because he wants to plan for a disability-free long life without brain atrophy, the world listens. Chris did his research about traumatic brain injuries, which can lead to degenerative brain disease or chronic traumatic encephalopathy (CTE). Trauma to the brain is just one cause of brain shrinkage (medically termed "brain atrophy").

I like to take a broader overview of the topic of brain atrophy, which looks at all of the factors that can lead to brain shrinkage including physical injuries to the brain from blows to the head.

The vast majority of cases of brain shrinkage do not come from physical injuries, but rather from medical illnesses. Many of them including many sports injuries are preventable, and I will deal with those points here.

Brain atrophy means a loss of brain cells, which causes a smaller brain. An MRI scan, which is available for a cost between $800 and $1000, will give information about the brain. The most sophisticated tool to depict the functioning of the brain may be the SPECT scan (ranging from $2000 to $2500).

What causes brain atrophy?

It is important to realize that a multitude of different factors can cause the same end result – brain atrophy. All of these factors work together causing brain atrophy and the more factors are at play the worse the outcome. So, let's review the various known causes of brain atrophy.

Diabetes

It has been known for a long time that diabetics can develop brain atrophy and dementia when their blood sugars are not well controlled. This leads to the formation of advanced glycation end products (AGEs).

Insulin and IGF-1, a factor produced by the liver in response to human growth hormone have been found to counter the development of brain atrophy in diabetics.

The key in patients with diabetes is a close control of blood sugars, best measured as the hemoglobin A1C blood test. At the 22nd Annual World Congress on Anti-Aging Medicine In Las Vegas (Dec. 10-14, 2014) Dr. Theodore Piliszek stated that the new normal range for hemoglobin A1C is 3.8 to 4.9%, quite a bit lower than the normally recommended values. Accepting the old values that proclaim that levels of 5.5 are still "normal" automatically puts you in a higher risk of developing brain atrophy and dementia.

Cardiovascular disease

What is good for the heart is good for the brain. That is what Dr. Perlmutter stated in his book. But the reverse is also true: if your cardiovascular system is sick, your brain gets sick!

Another investigator, Jack de la Torre published a paper showing how intimately connected heart function and brain function is.

Cardiovascular disease is a broad term and includes atrial fibrillation, blood clots in the coronary arteries or brain vessels (medically called "thrombotic events"), high and low blood pressure, heart failure, heart valve defects, low cardiac output, inflammation in the blood and a genetic marker, called Apo E, which is commonly associated with Alzheimer's disease.

The end result of any of these conditions will cause brain atrophy. Once a problem is identified, it is important that the patient is seeing the appropriate specialist who will take care of the risk factor in order to prevent brain atrophy.

Vitamin B deficiency

Some people are born with a certain degree of a methylation defect, a deficiency of certain enzymes, which prevents methylation of brain hormones and other metabolic products. This can lead to depression, schizophrenia, memory loss and - you guessed right - brain atrophy, which manifests itself as Alzheimer's disease or dementia.

By using the proper nutrients with high enough supplements of vitamin B2, B6 and B12 this biochemical process can be restored and brain atrophy can be prevented. Same is also a useful supplement that supports methylation leading to a normal brain metabolism. For a detailed

discussion about methylation defects read William Walsh's book, which explains this in detail (see references).

Obesity

The question is whether the "brain shrinks as the waist expands". The answer is a clear "yes". Researchers have found that the grey matter, which is responsible for our thinking and is in the frontal lobes of the brain, shrinks in obese people of all ages. The researchers found further that the grey matter shrunk in the temporal and parietal parts of the brain of people in middle and old age.

The key here is to cut out refined carbs (sweetened sodas, pasta, bread, sugar in any form), as they are the ones that cause obesity. This occurs by the liver metabolizing sugar and turning it into fat that is stored. Just by cutting out sugar and starchy foods both my wife and I lost 50 pounds each in 2001. It can be done, but it takes a bit of will power.

You may wonder how obesity can cause Alzheimer's: it is really the sugar from food getting metabolized into fatty acids by the liver causing obesity and hyperinsulinism; this in turn causes brain atrophy from damage to the blood vessels of the brain.

Smoking and alcoholic beverages

Smoking leads to brain atrophy by damaging the blood vessels that are supposed to supply the brain with nutrients. If blood vessels close off or there is hardening of the arteries, the blood flow to the brain is reduced, brain cells die, and brain atrophy develops.

Smoking also robs the body of vitamins, which slows down the brain cell function.

Alcohol is a nerve cell poison; it causes brain atrophy by directly damaging the brain cells (grey matter).

The results are memory loss, poor judgment, and problems planning one's future as well as loss of control with regard to emotions. This can lead to uncontrolled behavior, personality changes and problems with regard to inter-personal relationships.

Genetic factors

ApoE4 gene variant, which causes inherited Alzheimer's disease, causes a change of brain metabolism with deposits of a glue-like substance in the brain that damages nerve connections resulting in memory loss.

Researchers believe that ApoE4 is implicated in 20 to 25% of all Alzheimer's cases.

Despite this apparent negative story, there is hope by radically changing one's diet and taking supplements. Not every patient with one or two doses (alleles) of ApoE4 comes down with Alzheimer's.

What can you do to prevent brain atrophy?

Supplements: Take regular B complex vitamins (particularly B2, B3, B6, folic acid, B12), vitamin E and C, carnosine, acetyl-L-carnitine, boron, ginger, coenzyme Q-10 (or CoQ-10), curcumin, vinpocetine, zinc, grape seed extract, blueberry extract, Ashwaganda, glyceryl-phosphoryl-choline, Same, huperzine A and DMAE. All of these have been found to support brain function and often restore memory function. Unfortunately regular anti-Alzheimer's medications are not keeping their promise and on average just delay Alzheimer's by 3 to 6 months. For details how these supplements work see the previous section "Preserve your memory".

Omega-3 fatty acids including DHA: These essential fatty acids from fish oil are very useful as they are anti-inflammatory and help support the normal brain metabolism, particularly DHA. In a Feb. 2015 US study from the Rhode Island Hospital 193 Alzheimer's patients, 397 individuals with mild cognitive impairment and 229 normal individuals were followed for 5 years with MRI scans and cognitive tests every 6 months. 117 subjects were taking fish oil on a regular basis. The study showed a decline in gray matter in those who did not take fish oil and in carriers of the apolipoprotein E4 gene. The gray matter on the MRI scans and brain function measured with cognitive function tests were much better preserved in those who took fish oil supplements.

Resveratrol: This powerful antioxidant is an anti-aging supplement. It is preventing heart disease, hardening of the arteries and helps preserve brain function by keeping the brain vessels from getting clogged up. DHA and omega-3-fatty acids are helping in that regard as well.

Eat nuts: Nuts are healthy (provided you are not allergic to them); but just because you are allergic to one kind of nuts does not mean you are allergic to all of them. Often a person allergic to hazelnuts will not be allergic to Macadamia nuts, cashew nuts or walnuts. Nuts contain a mixture of essential fatty acids, blood vessel friendly, saturated fatty acids and minerals that are all brain supportive.

Exercise regularly: Whoever moves and exercises keeps the heart healthy and whatever keeps the heart healthy keeps the brain healthy as stated before.

Stress management and sleep (avoid chronic overstimulation of your brain): In our hectic society everything has to be instant, the expectations of managers are high, and the labor force is stressed. The fastest runner, the best player etc. is celebrated. The rest of us often feel like "underdogs", if we allow this type of thinking to rule ourselves. Use yoga, self-hypnosis, meditation, religious mediation and prayer to counter some of the stress from everyday life. We need some stress to get us going, but we do not need "distress". Dr. Hans Selye, the father of the general adaptation syndrome due to stress, gave a lecture about this topic in Hamilton, Ont. in 1977, which I attended. I vividly remember how he projected a picture of his skeleton showing bilateral hip replacements. He said that chronic stress could lead to arthritis. He had developed end stage arthritis in his hips and required total hip replacements on both sides. He wanted to illustrate that stress leads to physical consequences; it may be a heart attack in one person, a stroke in another, arthritis in a third. Constant overdrive has physical consequences.

Avoid sugar and starchy foods: I left this point as the last as it may be more difficult to understand. I started touching this topic under "obesity" above. An overload of refined carbs leads to an overstimulation of the pancreas pouring out insulin. Too much insulin (hyperinsulinemia) causes hormonal unbalance and leads to diabetes type 3, the more modern name for Alzheimer's. All starch is broken down by amylase into sugar, so essentially you get a sugar rush from any starchy food as well. Too much sugar in the blood oxidizes LDL cholesterol, which leads to inflammation in the body. The consequence of this are the following conditions: hardening of the arteries, strokes, heart attacks, Alzheimer's due to brain atrophy, arthritis, Parkinson's disease and cancer. I have blogged about these topics in many separate blogs in my anti-aging blog www.askdrray.com

Conclusion

I have reviewed how brain atrophy develops. There are a multitude of factors that over a lifetime can lead to brain atrophy. Repetitive head trauma from contact sports is only one reason; poor nutrition with too much sugar and starch and missing essential fatty acids (omega-3/DHA) is another potential cause. Add to this a lack of exercise, too much stress, alcohol and smoking and you covered most of the causes. Studies have shown that even when you carry the ApoE4 gene trait, only 30% will express it as supplements can suppress the expression of it, which is called epigenetic regulation. The key is prevention. Preserve your brain cells and prevent brain atrophy!

Alcohol will result in memory-loss later in life

Researchers found that heavy alcohol use in males during midlife paves the way to memory loss from dementia later in life.

I thought that this would be a good topic in order to review the effects of alcohol in general. Alcohol is a known cell poison, yet cardiologists keep on referring to the beneficial effects of that 1 glass of wine per day that will prolong your life. I will attempt to explain these diverse effects, where small amounts are supposed to be good for you while high amounts can be very damaging.

Review of the effects of alcohol

50% of the world population drinks alcohol, 10% to 20% have chronic alcoholism. In a Guardian news study in 2014 statistics were shown that an astounding 25% of Russian men die before reaching the age of 55, compared to only 7% of men in the United kingdom and less than 1% of men in the US. The study looked at the effects of consuming large amounts of vodka. There are about 10 million chronic alcoholics in the US. Chronic alcohol consumption leads to 100,000 deaths every year in the US. More than 50% of these deaths are from traffic accidents, the rest from medical problems caused by alcohol. Most of the alcohol gets detoxified through the liver cells and is metabolized into acetaldehyde. This involves the cytochrome P-450 system in the liver. This means that when narcotics, sedatives or psychoactive drugs are also taken the person will get into toxic levels sooner, because these medications are all metabolized through the same liver enzyme system as alcohol is. The mix takes longer to be detoxified, and this can lead to lethal overdoses that we hear about on the news all the time; hence the warning that you must not mix alcohol with drugs!

Alcohol is a cell and nerve poison. The most vulnerable organs in the body are the liver, brain, heart, pancreas, bone marrow and stomach. So, here are a number of conditions caused by drinking alcohol:

a) Anemia: When a person drinks heavily and regularly anemia shows up in a blood test. Alcohol has a toxic effect on the bone marrow, which interferes with the production of red blood cells. But certain vitamins required by the bone marrow to manufacture red blood cells are often also missing in the diet of an alcoholic, which contributes to anemia as well.

b) Cirrhosis: In 10% to 20% of heavy drinkers Cirrhosis of the liver will develope. With cirrhosis part of the liver cells get replaced by fibrotic tissue, and in advanced cases this can lead to a coma and death. Others are developing alcoholic hepatitis. This is an inflammation of the liver with fever and jaundice where the skin and eyeballs turn yellow. It is associated with severe abdominal pain.

c) Gastritis: Alcoholic gastritis is common, but often undetected. The affected individual may just have stomach pains for a few days, or vomit food and/or blood in addition. With continued use of alcohol it may turn chronic. Alcoholic gastritis can turn into gastric ulcers with massive bleeding that can lead to death.

d) Pancreatitis: The pancreas is a particularly vulnerable glandular tissue, which gets damaged by regular alcohol intake and with chronic alcohol intake gets partially replaced by fibrotic tissue causing the feared and painful chronic pancreatitis. This is a condition with vomiting and severe abdominal pains that can be unrelenting.

e) High blood pressure, seizures, dementia, depression, heart irregularities and nerve damage: You may ask yourself how all of these conditions would be reasonably dealt with one heading. The heading for this is “nerve damage”. Let me explain: The sympathetic nerve is very sensitive to alcohol toxicity and when the sympathetic nerve fibers are damaged, you will develop high blood pressure. You see your physician, get blood pressure medication, but the pressure is difficult to control, if you continue to drink alcoholic beverages. It does not make sense to just add blood pressure pills and hope that this will cure your problem. Seizures are due to direct nerve damage in the more sensitive parts of the brain, which will cause these areas to produce extra electrical activities, which we call seizures. Again, just treating with anti-seizure medications is not the solution. Avoidance of alcohol is the other part of the treatment schedule. Dementia from heavy alcohol use is due to direct nerve atrophy in the brain. Our brain shrinks normally 1.9% to 2.8% per decade, depending on which research papers you read. But in the presence of heavy drinking the frontal lobe of the brain is particularly vulnerable to brain shrinkage.

Mild and moderate drinkers did not suffer more frontal lobe shrinkage than abstainers did, but heavy drinkers had a 1.8-fold higher risk of frontal lobe shrinkage on average when compared to abstainers. It was calculated that alcohol had contributed 11.3% to that frontal lobe shrinkage.

Another toxic effect on the nerve tissue explains why depression would develop. The frontal brain contains most of the serotonin producing nerve cells. When serotonin-producing nerve fibers get damaged, the body does not produce enough serotonin to prevent depression from setting in; GABA producing cells often also get damaged, which causes anxiety. It's not good enough to just prescribe anxiolytic drugs for anxiety, to which the patient will get addicted or antidepressants for depression. The whole person needs to be treated, and abstinence from alcohol has to be part of the program.

Heart irregularities (atrial fibrillation, ventricular fibrillation) can be life-threatening complications due to the toxic effect of alcohol on the nerve fibers within the heart muscle. Emergency physicians are aware of the connection of these conditions to alcohol consumption. Some people's hearts are more sensitive to the effects of alcohol than others. The most common cause of temporary atrial fibrillation is excessive alcohol intake. It is caused the "holiday heart".

Finally there is the effect of alcohol on nerves in the body. This explains that heavy alcohol consumers can come down with painful pins-and-needles sensations in their hands and feet or with numbness or loss of muscle strength. When the parasympathetic nervous system is affected embarrassing incontinence or constipation can result. Erectile dysfunction in men who drink is also very common. Viagra and continuing to drink is not the solution.

f) Gout: This painful formation of uric acid crystals in joints can be precipitated in sensitive individuals by consuming alcohol in combination with eating large helpings of beef and other red meats. There may be a history of gout in the family. Treatment for this is to refrain from alcohol and avoid foods that are leading to uric acid production when ingested.

g) Cancer: When the body detoxifies alcohol in the liver, the breakdown product is acetaldehyde, which is a known cancer producing substance. A whole array of cancers are known, which come from heavy, chronic alcohol consumption: cancers in the mouth, larynx, esophagus, stomach, pancreas, liver and colorectal cancer have all been linked to excessive alcohol intake.

h) Cardiovascular disease: Heart attacks and strokes can be caused particularly by binging; it is thought that binging makes platelets from the blood more sticky so they clump together and cause blood clots, which in turn leads to heart attacks and strokes.

i) Infections: Alcohol weakens the immune system, which is another effect on the bone marrow similar to causing anemia, except that this is the toxic effect on the white blood cells and lymphocytes. Heavy alcohol consumers are more prone to pneumonia, to HIV, sexually transmitted diseases, and tuberculosis.

Cardiology view of preventative alcohol

Despite all of these hair raising toxic effects cardiologists have painted the rosy picture that 1 glass of wine for women and 2 glasses of wine for men per day will prevent heart disease. What is the true story here?

There are about 100 prospective studies that confirm that there is an inverse relationship between mild to moderate alcohol consumption and "heart attack, ischemic stroke, peripheral vascular disease, sudden cardiac death, and death from all cardiovascular causes". The reduction of risk in these various studies was persistent and consisted of a 20% to 45% risk reduction. Using blood tests investigators have found that this is because of an increase of HDL cholesterol, reducing blood clotting, making platelets less sticky and reducing inflammation as evidenced by a reduction of the C-reactive protein. Further research has pinpointed that it is the phenols and resveratrol that are contained in alcoholic beverages that are responsible for the beneficial effects. The bad news is that three or more glasses of wine do the opposite; so does binge drinking. Unless you are extremely disciplined and never increase your allowed limit (1 drink for women, 2 drinks for men) you will CAUSE heart disease rather than PREVENT it. Some people have a family history of breast cancer or colon cancer and they should avoid alcohol altogether; People coming from alcoholic families should also avoid alcohol altogether, because they cannot control their alcolhol consumption.

Conclusion

Where does this leave us with regard to prevention of heart attacks, strokes and hardening of the arteries in the legs (peripheral vascular disease)? If you are disciplined and stick to the limits, you could prevent 20% to 45% of cardiovascular risk. The brain study mentioned in the beginning of the blog would also confirm that there was no difference between dementia or brain shrinkage when mild to moderate drinkers were compared to abstainers over 10 years. What is not told by the wine industry is that

the same effects that prevent cardiovascular disease in mild to moderate drinkers can also be achieved by natural means: exercising regularly will raise your protective HDL cholesterol; taking ginkgo biloba, flax seed and omega-3 fatty acids thins your blood and the platelets are getting less sticky; omega-3 reduces inflammation and resveratrol elongates telomeres making you live longer. At the A4M conference in Las Vegas in December 2011 there were three speakers who pointed out that even small amounts of alcohol will poison mitochondria of your cells and interfere with normal hormone action. This was enough to make me join those who abstain from alcohol completely. One thing has not yet been investigated in long-term studies, namely how small effects of alcohol may affect the body over several decades and over an entire lifetime. Despite of all the promises of interest groups that red wine is a trendy drink for those interested in heart health, the fundamental long-term studies are missing. What does a guy do with a healthy heart and a brain that is not functioning too well? I just do not want to be the guinea pig in that worldwide study.

What alcohol does to you

Alcohol is being praised in the media for preventing heart attacks. But then we hear about alcoholic hepatitis and liver cirrhosis, both of which can be killer diseases. So, let us discuss what alcohol does to you.

Dr. Finnel pointed out that 7.9% of all emergency room visits in the US are due to alcohol related conditions. When the causes of deaths related to alcohol are listed, the top 8 causes are: cancer of the mouth and pharynx, alcohol abuse disorders, coronary heart disease causing heart attacks, cirrhosis of the liver, traffic accidents, poisonings, falls and intentional injuries. This is not what you read in the news. What you do read about is that one glass of red wine per day would be good for women and up to two glasses of red wine would be good for men to prevent heart attacks and strokes.

Bioflavonoids

It has been shown that it is the bioflavonoids and among those, in particular resveratrol, that are the active ingredients in red wine responsible for heart health. Resveratrol is a powerful antioxidant that protects the arteries from plaque. It is responsible for the cardio protective properties of red wine known as the "French paradox". Resveratrol is involved in at least 3 metabolism-stabilizing processes, so no wonder that you live longer whether you get resveratrol mixed in red wine or take it as a supplement from the health food store.

Toxicity of alcohol

Alcohol toxicity is a complex problem. According to the WHO 5.9% of all deaths worldwide are attributable to alcohol. In 2012 the WHO recorded that 7.6% of deaths in males were due to alcohol. In comparison, 4% of female deaths were due to alcohol. Toxicity comes from the breakdown product acetaldehyde. All cells convert alcohol into acetaldehyde, but liver cells are particularly well equipped to do this. Alcohol diffuses easily through all of the cell membranes and reaches every organ in the body. The toxicity of acetaldehyde is responsible for shutting down the mitochondria affecting the energy metabolism and causing cell death. Inflammation is caused by the immune system when it attempts to repair the damage.

So, what are the major problems of chronic alcohol consumption? These are the processes: First fat accumulation (steatosis), then chronic inflammation followed by necrosis (dying of cells) and fibrosis. An example of fibrosis is liver cirrhosis where liver cells are being replaced by non-functioning connective tissue cells.

Certain tissues are more susceptible to alcohol toxicity than others. As the concentration of alcohol is highest in tissues that are in direct contact with alcoholic drinks, cancers related to alcohol consumption develop in the oral cavity, pharynx, larynx, esophagus, and in the colon and rectum. The pancreas is particularly vulnerable to inflammation and fibrotic changes with subsequent degeneration into pancreatic cancer. The heart tissue and the arteries are very sensitive to alcohol; hypertension, heart attacks, stroke, cardiomyopathy and myocarditis as well as irregular heartbeats, called arrhythmias can develop from the effects of alcohol. The brain is also very sensitive to the toxic effects of alcohol. This causes major depression, personality changes with uncontrolled or violent behavior, car accidents and injuries. Kidney disease due to alcoholic nephropathy is another alcohol caused illness. 5% of breast cancers in northern Europe and North America are directly related to the toxic effects of alcohol. Finally, the liver being so active in detoxifying alcohol is affected by developing liver cirrhosis, which accounts for a lot of premature deaths at a relatively young age in the mid to late 50's.

Rusyn & Bataller mention in their textbook that literature exists which claims that 1 to 2 drinks per day would be useful for prevention of heart disease. But the observation of the authors is that people will not discipline themselves to stick to these limits and very quickly enter into the zone of alcohol toxicity. The authors further noted that with regard to causing any kind of cancer there is no safe lower limit;

the risk is directly proportional to the amount of alcohol consumed and the risk starts right above the zero point.

The pathologist has the last word

When I studied medicine at the University of Tübingen, Germany I attended lectures in the pathology department where Professor A. Bohle, M.D. demonstrated pathology findings of deceased patients. Dr. Bohle had a special interest in Mallory bodies. These are alcohol inclusion cysts within liver cells that can be stained with a bright red dye.

I will never forget when Prof. Bohle pointed out that the livers of this most diverse population, whose bodies we had the privilege to study as medical students, had a rate of 25% positive Mallory bodies. He wanted to impress on us as medical students to watch out for the alcoholics that are usually missed in general practice. Obviously 25% of the pathology population was affected by the consumption of alcohol. It was Prof. Bohle's hope that we could perhaps interfere on the primary care level before things went out of control. Many of these corpses belonged to traffic accidents that could have been prevented. Now seat belts and alcohol limits are standard, in 1968 when I attended to these lectures they were not.

Alcohol as an aging substance

Consistent use of alcohol on a regular basis will slow down cell metabolism and will also interfere with hormone production. The major effect of alcohol leads to poisoning of the mitochondria in multiple organs, which translates into faster aging and a shortened life expectancy. This in turn results in a change of appearance. An older person may look 5 to 10 years older than their chronological age.

50% of people above the age of 65 drink daily. Some more statistics: alcohol abuse in elderly men is 4-times higher than in elderly women. 5% to 10% of all dementia cases are related to alcohol abuse. About 15% of older adults are experiencing health risks from abusing alcohol. One more observation: about 90% of older adults are using medication and close to 100% of medications can adversely interact with alcohol.

Social pressure

These are the scientific facts, and then there is social pressure when you are invited to a party.

When you are young and invincible, do you care what the science says? You want to have a "good time" and not worry about consequences. The data about long-term exposure and a slowly increasing cancer risk is there. The wine industry will remind you that one drink for women and two drinks for men will protect you from heart attacks. They will withhold the cancer information from you, as they don't really want you to hear about that (yes, it's bad for their business!).

Can you have a good time at a party without drinking alcohol? Yes, you can. You can talk and you can listen; you are probably more with it than those who had too much to drink. I like mineral water and hold on to a glass of that.

There were three speakers at the 2011 Las Vegas conference who convinced me to join those who abstain from alcohol.

Socializing without alcohol is doable. You may at times miss it, but you can warm up even to a crowd that had a few drinks too much. It is about choice: we are free to choose what we want out of life. I believe that health comes first!

Conclusion

I have attempted to show you the toxic effects of alcohol. Although alcohol has played an important role in the social lives of millions over the centuries, it is becoming more apparent that alcohol is a cell poison and shortens our lives. The beneficial effect of the 1 or 2 drinks marketed by the beer and wine industry and some cardiologists does nothing to counter the threat in terms of a whole array of cancers at much smaller amounts of alcohol. Fortunately, resveratrol and omega-3 fatty acids as supplements as well as exercise will more than make up for the 1 or 2 drinks that you do not really need. And neither exercise, nor omega-3 fatty acids, nor resveratrol are cell poisons. The choice is yours!

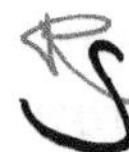

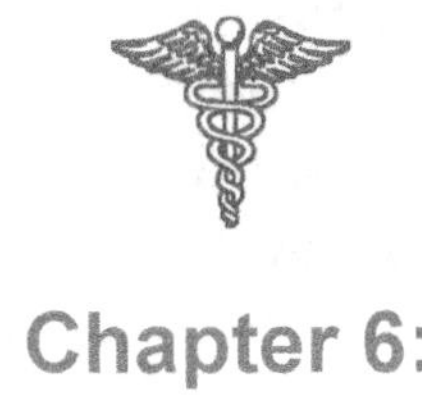

Chapter 6:

You Need a Healthy Heart

We all know how important our heart is for our survival. Here I like to explain how heart function can be measured. Then I need to debunk a myth: the "heart-healthy" low fat diet. Because this topic is so important I will delineate how the high carb/low fat myth makes you sick. And because we still have a lot of smokers among us, I need to talk about the fact that any kind of smoking is bad for you and that smoking is still a health hazard.

How to measure your heart function

Recently I came across a book by Dr. Steven Masley, cardiologist and fellow of the American Heart Association. The heart's function is to pump your blood reliably during your entire lifetime. It is a complicated organ, but it works well, if we treat it well. Western medicine has taught us that with complicated machinery and tests we can assess how the heart is doing. But until recently there was no reliable easier way to assess our cardiac health function. The purpose here is to summarize a three-pronged approach to measure your heart and blood vessel health. Dr. Masley

describes it in detail in his book. It is also important to FIRST see your doctor whether you are able to do the Bruce protocol (treadmill test, the third component below). If you neglect to be cleared by your doctor you run the risk of possibly getting angina pains or getting a heart attack from the treadmill test.

1. Carotid IMT or carotid intimal-medial thickness test: **You measure the degree to which there is hardening of the coronary arteries indirectly by measuring the thickness of the lining of the carotid arteries (carotid IMT or carotid intimal-medial thickness test). Dr. Masley has showed over a period of 10 years and more in many patients at his Health Center that there is a close correlation between the degree of coronary artery hardening and the degree of hardening of the carotid arteries. He stated that his research has shown that "90% of the time, the carotid arteries, the coronary arteries, and even the arteries of your legs all grow plaque at the same time". The gold standard for checking the condition of your coronary arteries is a heart catheterization as Dr. Masley explains. But he adds: "IMT testing should be the new gold standard for cardiovascular plaque testing. However, this is not yet the case. Despite its usefulness, 95% of doctors are not ordering this screening test for their patients. You can rest assured that this is a situation I am to change".**

2. A detailed lipid analysis called the VAP test: **this is a detailed laboratory test analyzing your lipid fractions (LDL, HDL, total cholesterol and VAP test). The buoyant HDL fraction, called HDL2 is the key to having a low risk for hardening of the arteries. HDL2 is large, fluffy and is designed to remove garbage from within the lining of the arteries. Also, the cholesterol ratio is another measurement for a low risk for hardening of the arteries when it is less**

than 3.0. The first two tests, the carotid IMT test and the VAP test, assess how much hardening of the arteries is present and when they are normal, there is a relative reassurance that nothing drastic - like a heart attack or stroke - should happen within the next 10 years. But this will only be the case if you keep up a regular exercise program and healthy food intake.

3. Bruce protocol (treadmill test): **The Bruce protocol (treadmill test) is often done by cardiologists, but is also offered in many gyms, where a trainer with experience in exercise physiology will do it. This functional test measuring cardiac output has been developed many decades back and has withstood the test of time. Here is an overview: as the slope of a treadmill and the speed of the belt are increased, the heart needs to do more work to maintain blood flow to your extremities and vital organs. The trainer or exercise physiologist measures the response of the heart activity in relation to the increase of the exercise load. A complicated formula allows calculating how much your maximal cardiac output is. This test has several variations and can be complicated to understand. Essentially, the higher the numbers you can create, the better. There are tables available where you can look up the various results of the VO2 max (maximal volume of oxygen consumption) from Bruce protocols and how they are interpreted.**

4. Treating abnormalities found with the three basic tests: **These are the necessary tools that tell you where you are in regard to your heart function. People with heart failure should not do this third test, because their heart muscle is too weak to sustain this demanding test. They would get heart failure, meaning that blood gets backed up into the lungs, and there could be severe breathing problems leading to a lack of oxygen (anoxia) in the heart tissue.**

This in turn can cause irregular heartbeats (fibrillation of the heart muscle) and a heart attack. Assume that the first two tests were within the normal limit for your age, and then the Bruce protocol would give you the maximum heart output at the peak level of your treadmill test. At this point you are measuring directly the cardiac output (what your heart is capable of pumping for you in a certain time unit). This measurement is what physicians call the VO2 max or maximal oxygen consumption. This is the best index for maximal heart capacity. If your levels are higher than normal, you have extra reserves with respect to your heart as a reserve for times when you need it. If this latter tolerance test shows poor results, it usually means that you were inactive and you would benefit from an exercise program. If the first test shows hardening of the arteries more than is appropriate for your age, you would need to look at your eating habits, particularly at the consumption of sugar and starchy foods as they cause lipids to rise. At the same time often the VAT values and the cholesterol ratio is off, meaning that you are eating the wrong foods and it shows in your blood test results as well.

5. Advice regarding diet, exercise and relaxation: Dr. Masley's book has several sections that explain what needs to be done when things are not normal. For instance, the author does not mince words when it comes to eating the right fats and cutting out sugar and starchy foods. For instance on page 199 there is a neat table that lists the fiber content of different foods. We need more fiber to slow down the absorption of sugary substances, which will minimize the insulin response following a meal. Dr. Masley also mentions that omega-3-fatty acids from fish and good seafood choices will balance the omega-6-fatty acids. It is unbalanced omega-6 fatty acids that activate the arachidonic acid pathway, which causes arthritis, inflammation and cancer. There are many more dietary recommendations, too numerous to repeat them all here. Suffice it to say, that molecularly distilled omega-3 fish oil, vitamin D 1,500 to 3000 Units daily, and magnesium supplements are all good for your heart. Vitamin K2 gets calcium out of your blood vessels and into the bone (100 to 200 micrograms per day). Other worthwhile supplements mentioned in the book are CoQ-10 (50 to 200 mg twice per day), but it would be wise to have blood levels drawn, which should be above 2.5mcg/ml to which the CoQ-10 intake could be titrated. Curcumin and Resveratrol are also recommended. Most of all, it seems that regular physical exercise such as a balanced gym program is the single most effective way to reverse hardening of the arteries, as measured by carotid IMT testing.

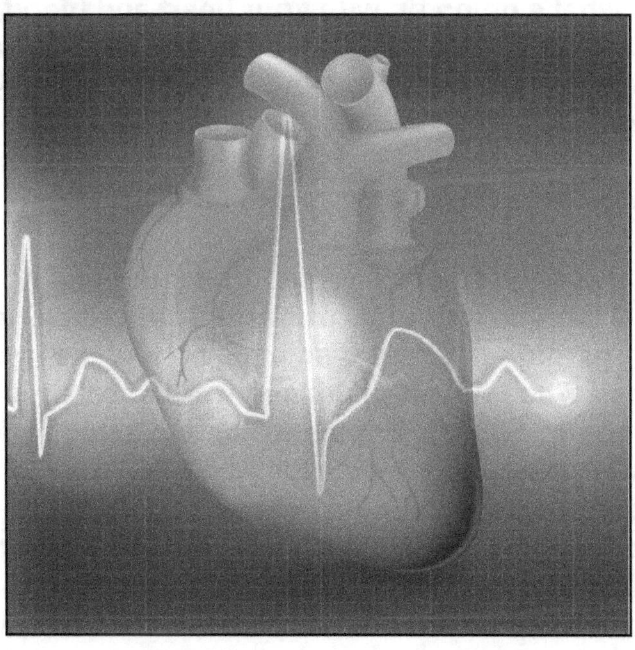

Conclusion

Times have changed. It used to be thought that our lives were following a one-way street downwards. During periods of malnutrition, lack of exercise, being sessile and abusing alcohol and drugs this may well be the case. However, we now know that fat deposits in arteries are reversible. Change to healthier food, start smoothies with organic vegetables in a blender, get going and walk, jog or use a gym to get regular exercise. Physical exercise reverses the fat deposits inside the lining of the arteries. The HDL-2 fraction rises and helps counteract the elevated LDL cholesterol. Even the mood of the person who exercises regularly becomes more stabilized. Using these simpler three tests, the physicians will not need the more complicated Thallium heart scans, or heart catheterization. These three tests described above are well worth being done every two years, so that you can monitor what's going on with your heart and blood vessels in general. After all heart disease is still the leading killer and close monitoring of our heart health will pay health dividends.

Forget the low-fat diet

The British Medical Journal (BMJ Publishing Group, James J DiNicolantonio) published a critical editorial review regarding the lack of science behind the low fat diet guidelines. The low fat guidelines were enacted in 1977 in the US and in 1983 in England. The devastating fact was that it was based only on a study of 2,467 men, and not a single female was included! There was no evidence of lower heart attacks in the low fat diet group when compared to the normal diet control. Yet the guidelines were the cause of the obesity and diabetes epidemic that followed and caused heart attacks and strokes. The myth about the low

fat diet persisted, but finally an article in the British Medical Journal exposed the falsity of this approach.

The BMJ Publishing Group re-traced all of the data that were available at the time of the decision in 1977. There were six randomized clinical trials with a mean duration of 5.4±3.5 years where low fat diet was compared to normal diet. The researchers found that the authorities that wrote the dietary recommendations for a low fat diet should have come to the conclusion that there was no statistical difference between the experimental group and the control group. The summary of the present re-analysis of the studies that were available to the US government in 1977 and to the UK government in 1983 was as follows: "There was no statistically significant relationship between dietary interventions and all-cause mortality."

It was noted that the all-cause mortality was identical in the experimental group and the control group (370 deaths in both groups). No significant difference of coronary heart disease (CHD) was observed between the low fat diet group and the control group.

There was no statistically significant difference in deaths from heart attacks. The reductions in mean serum cholesterol levels were significantly higher in the intervention groups; however, this did not result in measurable differences in mortality from CHD or all-cause mortality.

What is further troubling is that the six randomized studies that were the basis of all of these observations included only 2,467 men, but not a single woman. Yet the diet recommendations were made for both men and women alike.

The authors concluded "It seems incomprehensible that dietary advice was introduced for 220 million Americans and 56 million UK citizens given the contrary results from a small number of unhealthy men". And yet it was done! It

started people on a precarious course to an obesity and diabetes epidemic!

Dr. Robert Olson of St. Louis University warned Senator George McGovern that the studies did not support the dietary recommendations the Senator was about to announce. To this objection Senator McGovern replied: "Senators don't have the luxury that the research scientist does of waiting until every last shred of evidence is in".

There was very good evidence that a low fat diet did not change the rate of heart attacks and strokes. Yet the government committees in the US and in Great Britain did not consider this evidence. Other publications have examined the consequences of replacing saturated fats with carbs in the recommended low fat diets.

In a publication "The oiling of America" the following observations regarding low fat diets were made:

In processed foods low fat diet meant that more sugar was added to bring the saturated fat content down. This has detrimental effects on insulin sensitivity and causes type-2 diabetes on the long-term. Small LDL particles are increased and so are triglycerides, while HDL is reduced. Blood clot markers increase, weight increases, and obesity rates increase. Saturated fats were replaced with polyunsaturated fats of the omega-6 type from corn, soybean, safflower and cottonseed.

However, randomized controlled trials showed that when trans-fats and saturated fats were replaced with omega-6 polyunsaturated fats (without simultaneously increasing omega-3 fatty acids) increased death rates from heart attacks and strokes were found.

The Anti-Coronary Club trial showed that more people died from heart attacks when saturated fat was replaced by polyunsaturated fat.

The reason for the heart attack causing omega-6-fatty acids (from polyunsaturated fats) has been worked out

in several research papers between 2006 and 2012: they cause inflammation, cause cancer, weaken the immune system, lower the protective HDL cholesterol and increase the susceptibility of LDL cholesterol to be oxidized.

When saturated fat was replaced by polyunsaturated fatty acids (omega-6) the rates of breast cancer and prostate cancer increased.

This review ended with the statement that there is a lack of data supporting that a low fat diet helps prevent heart attacks and strokes. We have now clinical trials that numbered 347,747 participants. These trials showed that increased fat intake did not cause heart attacks. The women's health Initiative included 48,835 postmenopausal women showing that a low fat diet did not reduce cancer, and it also did not prevent heart attacks or strokes. All of this supports what has been summarized before in a critical review entitled "The Oiling of America".

The entire low-fat era has brought a public health disaster in its wake. A poorly done piece of research has not contributed to health, but to the upward spiral of health expenses. It has done nothing to keep a nation healthy, but everything to make a nation fat, sick, miserable and disabled. And now after decades we are trying to clean up a train wreck! It is a monumental task!

Conclusion

Enjoy saturated fat as it does not cause you harm. This does not mean that you start doling out a quart of melted butter over your vegetables. Cut out omega-6 fatty acids like oils from corn, soybean, safflower and cottonseed. Use virgin olive oil or coconut oil instead. Take regular supplements of omega-3 fatty acid (marine derived) to balance natural omega-6 fatty acids in turkey or chicken meat. You can eat cheese. If you are in the US, buy organic or imported cheeses from Europe where bovine growth hormone is illegal. Another source of beneficial fats comes from nuts; enjoy them! The only exception is peanuts. They do not have the same beneficial fats and are actually a legume.

It is most important to avoid sugar, honey, high fructose corn syrup and the currently fashionable agave syrup. There is no "healthy" maple syrup either. All of them have the nasty quality of oxidizing LDL cholesterol, which is the pre-stage for hardening of the arteries. The oxidized LDL cholesterol is incorporated into the plaques of arteries and leads to strokes and heart attacks. This also means that you must avoid all processed foods that contain sugar and high fructose corn syrup. It is important that you read labels on food products! Also, be aware that starchy foods (pasta, potatoes, cookies, bread, muffins etc.) turn into sugar within only 30 minutes in your digestive tract.

It is not that difficult to follow such diet recommendations. Lots of people have made changes. My wife and I have done this since 2001. We use stevia to replace sugar for sweetening (no calories, no effect on insulin). Do what's good for your body!

High carb/low fat myth makes you sick

If you are like most people, you probably still think that "healthy grains" like wheat are good for you and are "essential for a well balanced diet". Ever since Kellogg's introduced cereal for breakfast and the bagel was invented as a mid morning snack, the Agro Industry and the food industry have lobbied to have "healthy grains" in the food pyramid or on your plate. The very thought of "the daily bread" is deeply ingrained in our culture.

Other agencies like the Heart Foundation, the Academy of Nutrition and Dietetics (formerly "American Dietetic

Association") and the American Medical Association have reiterated this statement over and over until both the public and physicians accepted this as the truth. However, the scientific data does not support this point of view! It has been a myth! And unfortunately the consequences are not beneficial to your health.

We are gradually learning that there has been a big misinformation campaign going on as far back as 1984 and even earlier, when a consensus panel came up with revised normal values for cholesterol and we as the medical profession were told to treat high cholesterol levels much earlier and more aggressively than in the past with statins.

Big Pharma is still pushing for the use of cholesterol lowering statin. Now that I am retired for more than five years I can freely write about what is really going on. Much has been published abouth this but old habits in the public seem to persist.

I like to review the switch from the old school of thought that a high carb/low fat diet would be healthy to the new school of thought that a low carb/medium healthy fat diet is healthy. Before you panic, sit back, relax and read what I am saying.

A brief history of the high carb/low fat diet recommendation

The Framingham Heart Study is an ongoing study since 1948 that followed a large group of people for decades to sort out what causes heart attacks and strokes and how one could develop a program of prevention. This objective of the study was very noble and promising. However, as time went on the results from the Framingham Study that were published intermittently appeared to be more and more confusing.

First there was the lipid theory that was based on the observation that high lipids (called triglycerides) and high cholesterol in the blood would cause heart attacks and strokes. It was assumed that it must have been the fats in the diet that would have caused this. Based on this thinking the lipid theory of arteriosclerosis was formulated, a theory trying to explain how heart attacks would be caused.

If this theory were true, a lowering of the blood lipids and cholesterol should have lowered the rates of heart attacks and strokes. Many large trials were done and the statins were developed to lower cholesterol. All of this has not lowered the mortality rates from heart attacks and strokes, but instead of admitting that the researchers made a mistake, many are still doggedly holding on to the dogma of the lipid theory. The truth is that the lipid theory has not been proven to be true; the recommendation of a high carb/low fat diet has also not worked out to save lives by preventing heart attacks and strokes. In fact the opposite is true: older people with high cholesterol live longer and have less Alzheimer's disease than those with lower cholesterol levels in the blood as Dr. Perlmutter has explained in detail. Dr. Perlmutter mentioned a study from the Netherlands involving 724 individuals who on average were 89-years old that were followed for 10 years. Those with high cholesterol lived longer than those with low cholesterol, exactly the opposite of what the lipid theory predicted! Specifically, for each 39% increase in cholesterol there was a 15% decrease in risk of mortality. Think about it: the brain and the heart have LDL receptors on their cell surfaces for a reason. The reason is that both vital organs burn fat and need cholesterol to build up the membranes of the brain and heart cells.

Despite this compelling evidence Big Pharma is in denial and you will still find the lipid theory of arteriosclerosis heavily mentioned on the Internet as the only "valid"

explanation for how heart attacks and strokes would be caused.

Inflammation as the alternative explanation of arteriosclerosis

Since the mid 1990's the first reports surfaced to explain that about 50% of patients with normal cholesterol levels still develop heart attacks. In these patients the C-reactive protein, an inflammatory marker, was very high which indicated that it was likely an inflammatory process caused their illness.

Subsequently further research was able to show that the LDL cholesterol, when oxidized by sugar was responsible for clogged arteries in these patients. It also became apparent that diabetics have a much higher risk to develop heart attacks than patients with normal blood sugars. This led to the conclusion by different research teams that the lipid theory was wrong and needed to be abandoned.

Instead a new theory has developed that explains that heart attacks and strokes develop in patients where free radicals have damaged LDL cholesterol. This oxidizes LDL cholesterol and leads to hardening of the arteries (arteriosclerosis). Sugar from increased carbohydrate intake has a lot to do with this: it leads to glycation of protein causing advanced glycation end products (abbreviated as AGE's).

This is an appropriate name as "AGE" really is the cause of premature aging, of developing wrinkles, of getting premature hardening of arteries and having a 50-fold risk of free radical formation. This in turn will lead to more tissue aging. LDL used to be thought of as the "bad cholesterol". I myself have used that term in the past when explaining blood tests to my patients. Yes,I was wrong. LDL is now known to be the friendly and important transport form of cholesterol, which is sent from the liver to the brain and heart cells that need it for their metabolism. If LDL is oxidized, however, it becomes useless and the heart and brain cannot absorb cholesterol for membrane synthesis via the LDL receptors. The end result is that vital organs like the heart and the brain do not get enough oxygen and nutrients, which leads to heart attacks and strokes. The free radicals that are released from oxidized LDL cholesterol and that circulate in the blood cause an inflammatory response in the lining of the arteries all over the body, which you know as hardening of the arteries (medically termed "arteriosclerosis").

This may sound complicated, but all you need to remember is that sugar and starch consumption lead to accelerated hardening of arteries in your body, which causes heart attacks and strokes. It is that simple, but for donut lovers it will be hard to swallow.

Reassessment of what a heart healthy, brain friendly diet is

The above-mentioned research findings require a complete re-thinking of what a healthy diet would be. The villain turned out to NOT be saturated fat (meat, eggs, butter and avocado), but rather TRANS fat (margarine, hydrogenated polyunsaturated fatty acids) and the FDA made the right decision that trans fats have to go. Trans fat is full of free radicals oxidizing LDL cholesterol, which we just learnt is causing hardening of arteries. It is sugar and starches that turned out to be the main villain. Omega-6 fatty acids, found in safflower oil, sun flower oil, grape seed oil, corn oil and canola oil are bad for you also, as they lead to inflammation through the arachidonic acid system in the body. Conversely, flaxseed oil and omega-3 fatty acids (EPA and DHA) derived from fish oil are very protective and anti-inflammatory, as is olive oil and coconut oil. These latter two are anti-inflammatory monounsaturated fatty acids. Keep in mind that you want to change the ratio of omega-3 to omega-6 fatty acids more in the direction of omega-3 fatty acids, so that the ratio will be between 1:1 and 1:3. Most Americans are exposed to ratios of 1:8 to 1:16 (too many omega-6 fatty acids in fast food and processed foods), which leads to inflammation of the arteries as well.

The new "heart and brain healthy diet" consists of no refined carbs (sugar and starch), but about 45-50% complex carbs (organic vegetables like broccoli, spinach, cauliflower, Brussels sprouts, peppers, onions, garlic, peppers, Swiss chard, zucchini, asparagus etc.), 20 % protein and 30-35% saturated and other fats like omega-3 (1:3 mix with omega-6) fatty acids and monounsaturated fats (like olive oil or coconut oil).

According to Dr. Perlmutter you can even eat butter, lard and other animal fats provided they come from clean sources, not from animals that have been treated with antibiotics or bovine growth hormone. Dr. Perlmutter points out that even extreme diets like the Inuit diet with 80% saturated fat and 20% protein leads to longevity with healthy arteries. The patients who died in the many trials including the Framingham Heart Study did so, because of free radicals from sugar, starch and wheat. Wheat contains the addictive gliadin molecule (part of gluten), which makes people eat more sweets and starchy foods. The liver turns refined carbs into visceral fat deposits that in turn cause the release of cytokines like tumor necrosis factor alpha (TNF alpha) and COX-2 enzymes. These cause inflammation, heart attacks, strokes, arthritis and cancer.

Contrary to what Big Pharma wants you to know, cholesterol is an anti-inflammatory, LDL is a cholesterol transporter (provided it is not oxidized) and HDL is protective of hardening of the arteries as long as the "ratio of total cholesterol to HDL cholesterol" is less than 3.4 for males and less than 3.3 for females. This is the cholesterol risk ratio used by cardiologists to determine the risk of coronary artery disease. The average risk of this ratio for Americans is 5.0 for males and 4.4 for females. The ideal ratio to strive for is the ratio of 3.4 for males and 3.3 for women as explained in the Life Extension book.

Paradigm shift in causation of heart attacks and strokes, but also of cancer, and neurological diseases

As pointed out by Perlmutter there has been a paradigm shift in our thinking about what causes inflammation and what causes all of the major diseases including premature aging. Many physicians are not up to date in this new thinking although it has been in the medical literature since about 1995. In my colleagues' defense I like to say that they are busy people and they do not always have the time to do their continuing education. However, it is imperative that the public learns about this paradigm shift as it affects literally everyone. My YouTube video: Schilling, 2012 describes this new approach to medicine and how inflammation is the cause of many diseases. Now we are learning that there is a modified Zone diet or a modified Mediterranean diet that will prevent all these diseases. It is an anti-inflammatory, cholesterol containing, healthy fat rich diet without refined carbs, but containing ample complex carbs. At the same time it is a weight loss diet as cholesterol and fat in your diet stops the liver from producing lipids and triglycerides and helps you to lose weight. Critics will say that it sounds too good to be true, but I agree with Dr. Perlmutter and Dr. Davis, both of whom have provided ample evidence that it is true. Try some of their recipes. Just read Perlmutter's and Davis' books, where recipes are listed in the back part of their books. Or try the recipes I listed for one day below the conclusion. I have also published a book entitled "A Survivor's Guide To Successful Aging" through Amazon.com, which came out in March of 2014. You can find recipes for 1 week in the last chapter.

Conclusion

There has been a paradigm shift in the thinking of how hardening of the arteries is caused. Now it is known that an inflammatory process causes it. It is an overindulgence in sugar, starch and wheat products that causes the liver to produce lipids, cholesterol and leads to the "wheat belly" and the "grain brain". All of this causes cytokines to bring about an inflammatory reaction that affects the lining of arteries causing heart attacks, strokes, but also Parkinson's disease, MS, autism, asthma, arthritis, epilepsy, Lou Gehrig disease and Alzheimer's disease according to Dr. Perlmutter. The inflammation does not stop there. If you keep up the high carb/low fat diet, it will lead to various cancers. The solution is a diet high in healthy fats (I would call it a low carb/medium high healthy fat diet) as outlined above consisting of 30 to 35% healthy fat, 20% of protein and 45 to 50% of complex carbs, but none of the refined carbs. I have followed such a diet since 2001. I am enjoying that I can now eat a reasonable amount of healthy fats, which I was not aware of being allowed before I read Perlmutter's and Davis' books, but I continue with the antioxidant vitamins and anti-inflammatory supplements to prevent LDL oxidization. I hope that many of you can benefit from prevention, so you can enjoy a healthy life without being a victim of illness or disability.

Here is an example of what a day would look like nutritionally in terms of a breakfast, lunch and dinner

(Recipes by Christina Schilling):

Breakfast: Great Greens Omelette

(2 servings)
1 tablespoon olive oil or coconut oil
3 chopped green onions
3 cups spinach leaves or a mix of greens: kale, spinach, Swiss chard
1 red pepper cut into strips
3 eggs and 3 egg whites
2 tablespoons grated Parmigiano

In non-stick pan sauté green onion, greens and pepper strips in oil, stir eggs and egg whites and pour over the vegetables, sprinkle with Parmigiano. Cook on medium heat, till the egg mixture has started to set. Turn over and briefly let cook. Remove from pan, divide into two portions and sprinkle with a bit of salt (optional). Serve with salsa and guacamole.

Lunch: Oriental Salad

(2 servings)
1 small Sui choy cabbage (Napa cabbage)
2 cups mung bean sprouts
1 small daikon radish, shredded to yield 1 cup
1 red pepper, cut into thin slices
3 green onions, chopped
1 medium sized carrot, cut into matchstick size pieces
1 can sliced water chestnuts, rinsed.
Dressing: 2 tablespoons sesame oil,
2 tablespoons rice vinegar (light balsamic vinegar works too)
1-tablespoon Tamari soy sauce
1 tablespoon Thai sweet chilli sauce
1-teaspoon fresh grated ginger
3 tablespoons chopped fresh cilantro

Prepare all vegetables and put into salad bowl. Stir all dressing ingredients together and pour over vegetable mix. Stir gently, cover and refrigerate. This salad can be consumed immediately or kept refrigerated for a day. To complete the salad with a protein portion add your choice of 6 oz. cooked shrimp or the same quantity of cubed or sliced grilled chicken.

Dinner: Florentine Chicken
(2 servings)
1 large boneless chicken breast
1 tablespoon of chopped fresh basil-alternatively use 1 teaspoon dried basil
1 tablespoon grated Parmigiano
4 thin slices prosciutto
1 tablespoon olive oil
2 tomatoes- cut into halves
3 chopped green onions
2 cups baby spinach leaves
pinch of salt

Spread chicken breast flat and top it with the basil, Parmigiano and prosciutto slices. Fold into half and hold the stuffed chicken breast together at the edges with a toothpick or two. Heat olive oil in frying pan, add onion and tomato slices and put the chicken breast on top. Put lid on the pan, and cook at medium heat till the chicken is cooked through. If you test with a fork, the juices will be clear. Remove vegetables and chicken from pan, put on serving plate and keep warm. Remove toothpicks from meat, and cut chicken breast into two portions. Put spinach into pan and let the leaves wilt at medium heat(cover with lid). Put spinach on the side of the chicken and tomatoes, and sprinkle with a bit of salt.

Dessert after dinner: Berry Sorbet
(2 servings)
2 cups of deep frozen berries (strawberries, blueberries or a berry mix, no sugar added)
¾ cup of organic yogurt or goat's milk yogurt
a few drops of liquid stevia or small amount of powdered stevia-to taste.

Put into blender and process till smooth. You will have to open the blender jar to stir the contents in between. Serve with a dollop of whipped cream, —if desired.

Any kind of smoking is bad for you: Smoking still a health hazard

Recently new statistics came out that show that 48.8 million people in the US (19% of the population) still smoke. 22 % of the population is male, 17% female. Smoking is responsible for 20% of all deaths in the US (1 in 5 deaths). It is interesting to note that in the older age group (above the age of 65) only 8% are smoking, but 22 % of the 25 to 44 year old group is smoking. Among the American population Native Americans have the highest percentage of smokers (32% are smokers). 10% of Americans of Asian descend smoke. Blacks, Whites and Hispanics are placed in between them and the American Indians. Finally, people who can least afford it, (who are below the poverty level) have the highest percentage of smokers (29% of them smoke) while 18% of people above the poverty level smoke. Education seems to have a protective effect when it comes to smoking: of the least educated group of people 45% are smokers while only 5% with postgraduate education smoke.

Effects of cigarette smoke on the body

The mix of various ingredients in the smoke of cigarettes causes various parts of the body to react differently to these chemicals. Here is a rundown of diseases caused by smoking cigarettes.

1. Lung cancer: This is the most common cause of death in women who smoke, more common now than breast cancer. 90% of lung cancers in women are due to smoking. The same was true in males, but as a group they now smoke less than in the past.

2. Other cancers: Cervical cancer, kidney cancer, pancreatic cancer, bladder, esophageal, stomach, laryngeal, oral, and throat cancers are all caused by smoking. Recently acute myeloid leukemia, a cancer of the bone marrow has been added to the list of smoking related cancers.

3. Abdominal aortic aneurysm: As cigarette smoke destroys elastic tissue, it is no wonder that the loss of support of the wall of the aortic artery leads to the development of large pouches, which eventually rupture with a high mortality rate due to massive blood loss.

4. Infections of lungs and gums: Smokers are prone to infections of the lungs (pneumonia) and of the gums (periodontitis). Periodontitis is also related to heart attacks.

5. Chronic lung diseases: Emphysema, chronic bronchitis, and asthma are all related to smoking or made worst by it.

6. Cataracts: Lack of perfusion of the lens leads to premature cataract formation.

7. Coronary heart disease: Hardening of the coronary arteries, which leads to heart attacks, is very common in smokers causing heart attacks.

8. Reproduction: Reduced fertility in mothers, premature rupture of membranes with prematurely born babies; low birth weight; all this leads to higher infant mortality. Sudden infant death syndrome is found more frequently in children of smoking moms.

9. Intermittent claudication: After decades of smoking the larger arteries in the legs are hardening and not enough oxygen reaches the muscles to walk causing intermittent pausing to recover from the muscle aches. If it is feasible a cardiovascular surgeon may be able to do a bypass surgery to rescue the legs, often though this is not feasible and the patient's lower legs or an entire lower limb may have to be amputated.

10. Others: Osteoporosis is more common in smokers; poor eye sight develops due to age-related macular degeneration that sets in earlier and due to tobacco amblyopia, a toxic effect from tobacco on the optic nerve; hypothyroidism is aggravated by smoking and menopause occurs earlier.

What happens in the lung tissue in smokers?

A detailed rundown of the changes in the lung tissue as a result of exposure to cigarette smoke can be found in the Textbook of Respiratory Medicine under references. The various components of cigarette smoke lead to an activation of special white blood cells, called monocytes that after stimulation turn into tissue macrophages. In addition neutrophils (regular white blood cells) also get stimulated. Between them they produce cytokines and chemokines and the neutrophils secrete elastase that digests elastic tissue in the lungs. Breakdown products of the elastic tissue serve as a powerful stimulus to the immune system to mount an autoimmune response. After some time of being exposed to cigarette smoke the immune system considers part of the lining of the lungs as foreign and cytotoxic lymphocytes attack the lining of the air sacs (alveoli). Lung specialists consider chronic obstructive pulmonary disease (COPD or emphysema) to be an autoimmune disease.

The sad part is that when this condition has progressed far enough, even quitting smoking may be too late to stop the autoimmune disease by itself as the body has been sensitized and the immune system is convinced that the altered lung tissue should be attacked. Add to this that carcinogenic substances and toxins in cigarette smoke damage the DNA of all cells including the energy producing mitochondria, and the stage is set for the combination of chronic inflammation and the release of free radicals to cause all of the diseases mentioned above.

Quit smoking still important

It is extremely important to quit as soon as possible to avoid the full-fledged sensitization of the immune system against one's own lung tissue. Studies have shown that 36% of survivors of heart attacks will successfully quit, 21% of healthy men with a known risk of cardiovascular disease will quit when asked to do so and 8% of pregnant women will quit. When a physician examines a patient in the office and asks a smoker to quit smoking 2% of these smokers will respond and still not smoke 1 year after this doctor's visit. This may not sound like much, but it is an encouraging effect. Perhaps the most important fact is what I mentioned in the beginning of this section: the least educated group of people smoked the most (45%) while the most educated people smoked the least (5% of people with a postgraduate education). My hope is that the Internet and other educational media will contribute to education

and convince people how important prevention is, which will convince people to quit on their own simply because it makes sense.

Pharmacological assistance to quit smoking

Nicotine replacement therapy can involve any of nicotine polacrilex gum, transdermal nicotine patches, nicotine nasal spray, the nicotine inhaler or nicotine lozenges. If you smoke, discuss with your doctor what may be best to use in your case to assist you to quit. Typically one of these products is used for 3 to 6 months.

Bupropion is an antidepressant with a nicotinic acetylcholine receptor affinity. Bupropion is useful to help with the withdrawal from nicotine addiction, which occurs in depressed or non-depressed people. It strictly has to do with the stimulation of the nicotinic acetylcholine receptor. Typically the dose is 150 mg of a sustained released bupropion tablet per day for 7 days prior to stopping smoking, then at 300 mg (two 150-mg sustained-release doses) per day for the next 6 to 12 weeks. 44% quit at 7 weeks versus 19% of controls. A newer nicotine partial receptor stimulator, varenicline, has been compared to bupropion. It was slightly more effective in helping people to get off cigarettes. Varenicline is started at a dose of 0.5 mg per day for 3 days, then 0.5 mg twice daily for 4 days, followed by a maintenance dose of 1 mg twice daily. If nausea is a problem, lower doses can be used. Varenicline has been approved for a 3-month period with an option of a second 3-month period, if relapse occurs. Discuss with your doctor what is best for you.

A combination therapy of bupropion and nicotine patch was more effective than either one alone according to the Textbook of Respiratory Medicine.

Will power, hypnotherapy

Hypnotherapy to quit smoking has been popular, but is not as effective as it is often claimed. Will power, measured by the "placebo" response is quite effective given the fact that nicotine is very addictive and yet 19% in the placebo group were able to quit on their own. Varenicline treatment for 12 weeks produced abstinence for 9 to 52 weeks and was compared to bupropion and placebo. The abstinence rates were 23%, 15%, and 10% for varenicline, bupropion, and placebo. This means that will power was still 2/3 as effective as bupropion and 43% as effective as varenicline. Don't underestimate will power!

Conclusion

The best scenario is to never start smoking; the second best is to quit as soon as possible. Unfortunately, the third scenario of continuing to smoke is still very prevalent worldwide. I have seen the damage done first hand in practicing medicine, which motivated me to never smoke. But I am aware of the difficulties of quitting because of the highly addictive nature of cigarette smoking. Where is the support from governments on this? The problem is that the government benefits from taxation of cigarettes. Nevertheless it is laudable that there are government sites through the CDC to help you quit smoking. There are several private websites that are useful too.

In the end we are all responsible for our own health. If you are presently smoking, psych yourself up for the day that you will quit. Quitting means, that you are deciding actively to live longer. Studies have shown that it takes often several attempts before you eventually quit successfully.

Smoking e-cigarettes of no benefit

Electronic cigarettes (e-cigarettes) were invented to help people get away from the carcinogenic content of real cigarettes and they were thought to help people in the process to quit smoking as well.

In the October 2014 issue of the BC Medical Journal a review article is entitled: "Electronic cigarettes: Do we know the benefits vs. the risks?" In it Dr. Roy Purssell, the Chair of the Emergency Medical Services Committee in BC, Canada reviewed the literature about e-cigarettes. He pointed out that several studies have shown that the number of cigarettes used may have declined with the use of e-cigarettes, but the quitting rate on e-cigarettes is not higher than quitting conventional cigarettes.

Why were e-cigarettes developed?

Originally they were marketed as an alternative to cigarette smoking with the thought that they would only contain the nicotine, but not the myriad of cancer producing chemicals. However, studies now show that this is not the case. As explained earlier people use e-cigarettes, but they often still smoke real cigarettes on the side, in effect just reducing the number of cigarettes smoked per day. Says Dr. Purssell: "Reducing the number of cigarettes smoked per day is much less effective than quitting entirely for avoiding the risks of premature death from all smoking-related causes of death". The US Department of Health and Human Services came to a similar conclusion in 2014.

Chemical composition of e-cigarettes

E-cigarettes are battery-operated vaporizers that give you the feel of smoking a tobacco cigarette. The container inside the e-cigarette can be refilled with "e-juice" that can be bought through the Internet. The liquid contains highly concentrated nicotine, propylene glycol, glycerin, and flavorings (you can choose from cinnamon to cherry flavor and more). The liquid is vaporized by a heating element and the vapor is inhaled. No long-term experiments are available at this time with regard to the safety of these inhaled chemicals in humans. Only short-term experiments are behind the FDA's declaration that propylene glycol would be "generally recognized as safe" (GRAS) as a food additive. But there is still a difference between inhaling and ingesting propylene glycol, and the same is true for glycerin.

The manufacturers of e-liquid (or e-juice) always put this disclaimer on their products: "Warning: Always keep e-cigarette liquid in a safe place and out of reach from children and pets. Nicotine in its pure form is a poison, and can cause harm if ingested by a child."

Toxic effects of e-juice (e-liquid)

From September 2010 to February 2014 there were 2405 reports to the poison control centers in the US about e-cigarette exposures. In the month of February 2013 there were 70 calls, in February of 2014 there were 215 calls, a 300% increase. More than 50% of these cases involved young children.

In BC, according to Dr. Purssell the Drug and Poison Information Centre received 70 calls between July 1, 2013 and June 30, 2014. 50% of these involved children who were younger than 4 years old. There was no case of serious toxicity. If, however, enough fluid is swallowed, there can be deaths from nicotine overdose, particularly in children and in pets. Seizures can be caused by nicotine overdoses and poisoning of the breathing center in the brain stem.

Nicotine is highly addictive. In children and in adolescents nicotine has a negative effect on brain development. The Minnesota Poison Control Center, reported poisoning incidences with e-juice that was swallowed by young children and it also reported about adolescents who overdosed on e-cigarettes.

It appears that the nervous system is more sensitive for toxic effects of nicotine at a younger age.

Regulations of e-cigarettes

At this point e-cigarettes are illegal because the FDA is still examining the pros and the cons. The situation in Canada is similar: Under the Canadian Food and Drugs Act regulations it is currently illegal to sell e-cigarettes containing nicotine. The international Union against Tuberculosis and Lung Disease has issued a position statement saying that its preferred opinion is to regulate e-cigarettes as tobacco products. The UK will be following this advice.

Dr. Purssell commented: "This is a reasonable course of action for a product that delivers a highly addictive substance with negative effects on brain development and can cause serious poisoning."

While the Internet merchants are busy marketing these products, it is important that the legislators around the globe take swift action to draft policies and regulations now to protect children and adolescents.

Conclusion

In conclusion it can be stated that smoking e-cigarettes will not have any benefits whatsoever. Smokers still smoke, as the addictive substance (nicotine) in e-cigarettes undermines their efforts to quit. It may be true that they

are not exposing themselves to lung cancers as much as those who puff away on regular cigarettes, but instead their cardiovascular system is exposed to the nicotine that causes heart attacks and strokes. It sounds very sobering that trading e-cigarettes for tobacco cigarettes is just trading one cause of unnecessary death (lung cancer) for another one (strokes and heart attacks).

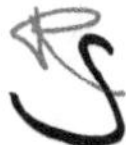

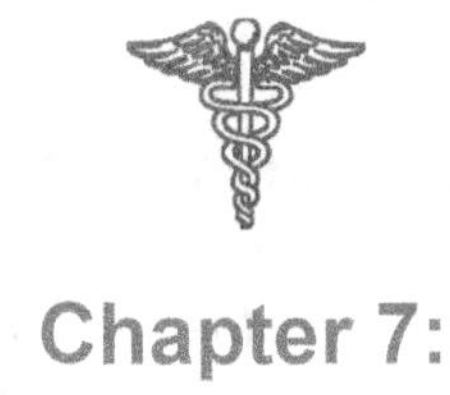

Chapter 7:

Why Food Matters

In the following chapter I will briefly review the various food components. The Mediterranean diet without sugar and pasta is what is now seen to be one of the healthiest diets. Part of the Mediterranean diet means that food is prepared with olive oil, which by itself is worth writing about.

We all have eating habits that can be a result of our upbringing and our cultural background, and there are dietary habits during the holidays that make a mess of any sensible eating. With the description of various foods there are the aspects about foods containing wheat. More and more people seem to suffer from sensitivity to wheat, and celiac disease has increased significantly compared to several decades ago. Could gluten have anything to do with our appetites? I will also review why sugar and starchy foods age us faster. This brings us to sugar substitutes; my favorite one is stevia. Eating out is always an issue, and a review of this will follow. A few other food-related issues like probiotics, olive oil, pure water and food safety are completing the chapter.

Yes, what we eat matters

Whoever has seen or heard of the movie "Super Size Me", released in 2004 will know that eating McDonald's food every day cannot be healthy. Too much fat, too many carbs, too many calories, a lack of fresh vegetables and fruit!

Anti-oxidant vitamins are contained in fruit and vegetables. They will help the mitochondria, our energy packages mentioned above to work under optimal conditions. However, apart from having balanced meals as described below we would do well to take a multitude of vitamins, antioxidants and minerals just to limit the damaging effect of free radicals attacking our bodies (including the mitochondria) every day.

I believe that the best diet is one that sticks close to the natural diet of those who live long, fulfilled lives and have lots of energy until a ripe old age. The population of Okinawa comes to mind as described by Willcox et al. in 2001. The Mediterranean diet is another example.

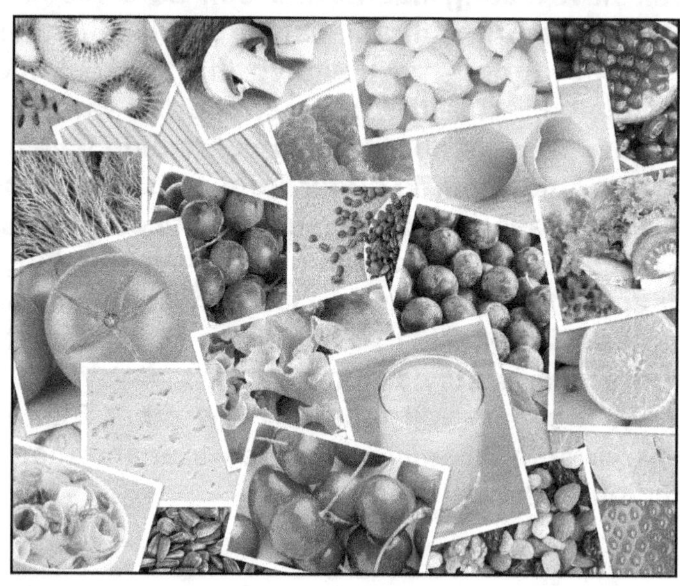

Protein Foods

We need protein to supply us with amino acids that are the building blocks of our own protein (muscles, all cells, but also many brain hormones, which are made from amino acids). Lean chicken, Turkey meat, pork, lamb, bison and grass fed beef come to mind. One author, Dr. Sears points out in his publications that protein helpings should not exceed the size of the palm of our hand. That goes for thickness as well!

The fat factor

We need essential fatty acids that are contained in fish and in fish oil supplements. They give us omega-3 fatty acids and DHT, which is essential for our brain cell metabolism. Omega-3 fatty acids are heart protective as well.

Extra virgin olive oil is a healthy oil that has substances in it that rejuvenate the lining of the arterial walls and prevents heart attacks and strokes. Two tablespoons of olive oil per person per day seems to be the magic number, which gives you the best health benefit.

Here are a few rules about fat to remember.

The do's and don'ts about fat intake

To make sensible and healthy choices you do not need a degree in nutrition. All you have to do is:

1. Read the labels and ingredient lists.

2. Avoid products, which contain hydrogenated or partially hydrogenated fats.

3. Eat one food per day, which contains omega-3 fats. (If you do not like fish, take three to six capsules of molecularly distilled fish oil.)

4. Use some monounsaturated fats like olive oil or coconut oil.

5. Aim for between 20 and 30% of fat content as part of your daily caloric consumption. Do not exceed the 30% mark. This means that you will look for fat amounts of 18% to 24% in cheeses and for 2% cottage cheese for snacking and also for low fat yoghurt.

With these simple guidelines, fat will be your nutritional ally and not an enemy.

Carbs

Glycemic index

The glycemic index helps us to understand which foods we should seek and which foods we should avoid. The glycemic response is derived from the height of the blood sugar level response that occurs when pure sugar is absorbed by the gut into the blood stream. This blood sugar level response was established as the norm and was arbitrarily given a value of 100%. Any other carbohydrate, which is less refined than sugar leads to a lesser response as the sugar level after absorption is less. Here is a table that lists the high glycemic index foods:

High GI foods that you should avoid (modified from pages 99/100, Willcox et al. 2001):

HIGH (>70%) GLYCEMIC INDEX FOODS TO AVOID					
FOOD TYPE	GI (%)	FOOD TYPE	GI (%)	FOOD TYPE	GI (%)
DOUGHNUT	76	BREAKFAST CERIAL:	FROM	GLUCOSE	100
CORN CHIPS	74	CHEERIOS, CORN	70 to	HONEY	87
SHORT WHITE GRAIN	72	BRAN/FLAKES, CRISPIX,	80	SUCROSE/SUGAR	75
WATER MELON	72	RICE KRISPIES, R. BRAN,		DATES	100
AUNT JEMIMA WAFFLES	76	SHREDDED WHEAT		COOKIES	76
WHITE BAGEL	72	INSTANT RICE	80	MALTOSE	105
WHITE BREAD	70	TAPIOCA WITH MILK	81	MSHD. POTATO	70

It is generally accepted that a low glycemic index is up to 55%, a medium index from 56 to 70% and a high index above 70%. Low and medium GI foods are recommendable; the high GI foods should be avoided. The above table gives you a flavor of what to avoid. These are the foods that make your insulin level spike after a meal, but between meals lead to a sugar level slump called reactive hypoglycemia. This is like a roller coaster ride for your metabolism. Now that you know which foods to avoid, what are the foods that are recommended?

They are the foods that will not cause the pancreas to produce an overabundance of insulin. So, they would also be the foods that diabetics could eat. Below I have summarized them in a table (modified from Willcox et al. 2001):

Newer research has shown that high glycemic foods including sugar and high fructose corn syrup oxidize LDL cholesterol, which causes atheromatous plaques in arteries; these calcify subsequently causing hardening of the arteries, which in turn leads to heart attacks and strokes. It is therefore a matter of life and death to stick to low glycemic foods to prevent this from happening. I have explained this in more detail in my recent book, published 2014.

LOW (<55%) AND MEDIUM (55-70%) GLYCEMIC INDEX FOODS RECOMMENED					
FOOD TYPE	GI (%)	FOOD TYPE	GI (%)	FOOD TYPE	GI (%)
FRUCTOSE	20	CHERRIES	22	SWEET POTATOES	50
AGAVE NECTAR 1TBSP.	11	RAISINS	65	TOMATOES	38
STRAWBERRY JAM 1TBSP.	51	STRAWBERRIES	32	CHICKPEAS	36
SPLENDA/OTHER ARTIF. SWEETENERS	0-2	APPLES	38	LEGUMES BEANS, LENTILS	29-36
BRAN MUFFIN	60	ORANGES	40	SOYBEANS	15
BROWN RICE	55	PEARS	45	YOGHURT PLAIN	35
CHEESE TORTELLIINI	50	MANGOS	55	WHOLE MILK	27
MEAT RAVIOLI	39	KIWIS	52	ICE-CREAM	37-61
WHOLE GRAIN BREAD	40-50	GRAPEFRUITS	26	MACARONI CHEESE	64
PUMPERNICKEL 1SLC.	41	GREEN PEAS	51	GR. LF. VEGETABLES	0-15
PINEAPPLE	66	LONG W. GRAIN	44	BARLEY PEARLED	25

Holiday binges - eat now, repent later

Countless blogs have been written about gaining pounds with holiday food. This is not my topic here. I am looking at the medical evidence of what is happening to our bodies, some of which is permanent. I like to focus on the gallbladder, blood pressure, heart function and gout. I will provide little clinical vignettes that make my points clear.

Gallbladder disease

Many patients are unaware that their gallbladder has developed stones that accumulate over several years, perhaps even several decades. But, if infection sets in there is an acute flare-up of gallbladder pain, which can be excruciating. Also, when one of the stones is transported into the gallbladder duct, there is a sudden colicky pain similar to labor pains. In cases where the migrating stone blocks the common bile duct, the patient can get jaundiced and the pancreatic juice can get backed up leading to an acute pancreatitis.

What does that have to do with overindulging during a Thanksgiving meal? Fatty sauces, ham, and gravy can all lead to more cholesterol deposits in the gallbladder and make stones larger. Add to this a rich dessert with ice cream and a dollop of whipped cream and you've got yourself a fairly fatty feast. So, this one fatty meal can make a difference by bringing on symptoms of a previously undiagnosed condition, and you spend hours in an emergency room of a hospital.

The scenario could look like this case:

Fred is a 40-year-old teacher, somewhat overweight who enjoyed a holiday meal at his parent's place for Thanksgiving. His health has been good with no surgeries. Following the turkey dinner, which he enjoyed, he noticed right upper abdominal pain, and he started to vomit. As the pain did not improve, his parents called an ambulance that brought him to the local hospital. The emergency physician said that he was concerned about Fred's gallbladder. He ordered a CT scan and this showed multiple stones with one of the stones being stuck in the cystic duct. Despite pain medication and bed rest the situation did not resolve (the stone did not pass). A surgeon was called in and a laparoscopic cholecystectomy was performed (removal of the gallbladder through a pin hole). Fred recovered within only 3 days and could return to teaching. The fatty food of the Thanksgiving dinner was only the tip of the iceberg in this case. The fact that there have been many pre-existing gallbladder stones tells us that this patient had the chronic habit to eat foods with too much fat and cholesterol; but sweets and carbs were also converted in the liver into fatty substances that made their way into his bile. The end result: gall stones formed out of the bile that was supersaturated with cholesterol; the gallbladder needed removal.

High blood pressure

Extra salt intake leads to an elevation of blood pressure. If a person has borderline high blood pressure, the extra salt intake from holiday meals can get the blood pressure out of control, and this in turn can cause a stroke (typically a hemorrhagic stroke) or is a strain to the heart leading to a heart attack or to congestive heart failure.

Janice is a 50-year-old janitor who has had problems with borderline high blood pressure readings. Normally her blood pressure was 140 over 90, and when she watched her salt intake it would go down to 125 over 80. She bought a blood pressure monitoring device, just so she could measure her own blood pressure at home. Following the Thanksgiving turkey dinner she noticed that she developed fullness in her head and a headache, and her face looked flushed. She took her blood pressure and got a reading of 160 over 100. It had never been that high. When she saw her doctor he asked her what she had for Thanksgiving dinner. She reported that she sat together with friends and had potato chips with dip and drank some red wine with it. Next for the meal she enjoyed the roasted, brined turkey and ham. Yes, she did add some more salt to the mashed potatoes too.

The doctor found her blood pressure to be 165 over 100. He explained to her that she needed to go on a DASH diet, which is low in salt. He also started her on blood pressure pills. With a sensible diet and other improved lifestyle habits it is conceivable that Janet may be able to get back to normal blood pressure readings.

Heart attack following turkey dinner

When working as an intern in teaching hospitals of McMaster University of Hamilton/Ont. during my training in 1975 to 1978 I noticed a strange correlation between holidays like Thanksgiving and Christmas and intensive care unit admissions with acute heart attacks. Later a formal study was published that there is indeed such a correlation between consuming a big meal with fat, salt and refined carbs and the development of a heart attack.

This does not develop without prior silent conditions like high triglycerides, high cholesterol and insulin resistance leading to inflammatory substances circulating in the blood. The C-reactive protein and a fasting insulin level have emerged as a useful monitoring device. Both should be low, or the person is at a higher risk of developing a heart attack.

Add to this a festive, large meal and you got troubles at your hand like in the next case:

Joan is a 62-year-old high school principal who developed chest pain within 2 hours after having enjoyed her Christmas dinner. She was known to have high cholesterol levels for about 5 years and she had been taking statins for 4 years as diet alone did not control the condition. But she loved food in general and was about 20 pounds overweight. The doctor had discussed exercise with her, but she felt too busy doing other things. Now all of this came back to her as she was recovering in a hospital bed from an emergency stent procedure. They had to insert two stents to overcome narrowing of the coronary arteries. She was now pain free and felt that she needed to do something about her lifestyle. She would see a dietitian and record her weights daily. She wanted to loose 20 pounds and yes, she wanted to start mild exercise when her doctor allowed it and gradually build it up to a maintenance program.

Gout attack following rich meal

It is known since the Middle Ages that feasting on a large meal of beef combined with lots of beer or wine can cause a gout attack. Gout at this time was known as a disease of the affluent. Henry VIII suffered from gout, and probably a lot more of his well-to-do contemporaries. The poor obviously could not afford big feasts. Today we know that purines are the end product of meats, and they get excreted through the kidneys. However, alcohol prevents the purines to be excreted in the urine so that uric acid levels exceed a certain limit beyond which uric acid crystals are precipitated in soft tissues around joints. This condition is quite painful and will often send a patient to the emergency room.

The following case will illustrate this:

Carl, a 45-year-old sales person suddenly developed excruciating pain and swelling in his left big toe. He went to the emergency room of the closest hospital. After some tests he was told that he had come down with acute gout. His blood tests showed a high uric acid level and biopsy samples from the left big toe also revealed uric acid crystals. With the help of colchicine and allopurinol things turned back to normal within 3 days.

The gout episode occurred just 4 hours after his holiday meal consisting of a few beers and copious amounts of turkey meat. He also is almost addicted to soft drinks, which are sweetened with high fructose corn syrup, and he consumes them freely throughout the day.

It is known that sugar from soft drinks make a person 85% more prone to develop gout than a person who uses diet drinks or water ("Gout leaflet" under References). But diet drinks are another story: do you really need aspartame? As mentioned earlier, it's a lousy idea! So, skip those diet drinks if you value your health at all.

Here is a diet sheet for Carl to prevent his next gout attack ("Gout diet sheet" under References).

Conclusion

Who would have thought in the past that food could be a dangerous substance with the potential of making us sick? But this is exactly what I wanted to point out in this section. Of course, it does not stop at holidays where we tend to eat more than what we normally eat. It pays dividends watching what we consume even in the days between feasts. For instance a DASH diet is a good idea for those of us who may have developed borderline high blood pressure. Avoiding excessive red meat is a good idea for prevention of heart attacks and strokes, as your cholesterol stays lower. Avoiding soft drinks with sugar and fructose is good prevention for avoiding obesity, cancer, heart attacks and strokes. Get the greens going (vegetables, salads etc.) to live longer without disabilities.

Gluten sensitivity

A report about gluten free food is circulating in the media. It points out that gluten-free food is not as healthy as advertising wants you to believe.

Wheat is the source of gluten, so rice, potato, corn and sugar are used to replace wheat. Corn is deficient in niacin leading to B3 deficiency; and the amino acids lysine and tryptophan (missing in corn) are needed for production of serotonin in the brain, which prevents you from getting depressed.

Gluten-free food is a special form of processed food. Any processed food is not as good as natural food that you buy from the periphery of the grocery store.

So, what do we know about gluten sensitivity?

Causes of increased diagnosis of gluten sensitivity

Only 1% of people are gluten sensitive at this point. Just 30 years ago this number was 0.025%. 10 years ago 0.04% of people were thought to have gluten sensitivity. The difference may be due to improved sensitivity of the testing methods. But another factor is the new wheat, called Clearfield wheat, which was obtained through chemically forced hybridization of wheat resulting in significant genetic modifications from the original wheat that our grandparents consumed. This type of wheat is now grown all over the world. Clearfield wheat has a significantly higher percentage of gluten, which likely contributes to the increased gluten sensitivity in the population at large and particularly among patients with irritable bowel syndrome (IBS).

Irritable bowel syndrome and other food sensitivities

According to Rakel's textbook "Integrative Therapy" 4 to 5% of patients with irritable bowel syndrome (IBS) have true gluten intolerance (celiac disease). In the general population (without IBS) the gluten sensitivity percentage

is less than ¼ of that. Sensitivity to food is not all about gluten, even though gluten is currently in the spotlight. Lactose intolerance in the US is found in 25% of all adults and in 35% to 45% of IBS patients. Another common food sensitivity is fructose and sorbitol intolerance, which occurs in about 40% of patients with IBS and about the same percentage in non-IBS controls. This means that if you leave out sorbitol and fructose, about 40% of people will find relief from abdominal cramps or bloating. A common item that people chew on is sorbitol-containing chewing gum. If this type of chewing gum is eliminated, 40% of people will feel better in their gut. The irony is that people could still chew gum with xylitol instead of sorbitol, if they are allergic to sorbitol. So, keep in mind that the majority of people with food sensitivities do not have gluten sensitivity, but lactose intolerance and allergies to fructose and sorbitol.

Other manifestations of celiac disease

Celiac disease is not only a disease that manifests itself as a skin rash (as originally described in celiac patients). It is responsible for a significant amount of ADHD (attention deficit hyperactivity syndrome) or ADD (attention deficit syndrome) and can even cause Parkinson's disease. It stands to reason that these conditions can be improved with an appropriate diet.

Gluten-free foods often contain problematic replacements

When you go to a grocery store or health food store and look at their gluten free shelves, they offer you an array of products like gluten-free bread and bakery items, cereals, cookies, pastas and many other processed foods.

As explained above, wheat is the main source of gluten and when you replace it, the substitutes are rice, tapioca starch, quinoa, potato, corn and sugar. We already pointed out some deficiencies of corn. There are also concerns of toxicities as in rice, as some sources can be contaminated by arsenic. As the majority of people with food sensitivities are allergic to milk sugar (lactose), fructose and sorbitol, these items have to be screened carefully by reading all of the details on the food labels of the products. If you suspect other food allergies, see your primary care physician for testing for these allergens and also have several of the gluten sensitivity tests done as listed under references. If the gluten sensitivity tests are all negative, you only need to pay attention to milk sugar, fructose and sorbitol, particularly, if you have been diagnosed with IBS.

Hidden sugar and starch content of gluten-free food

What has not been mentioned so far is the sugar and starch content in processed gluten free foods, which eventually leads to higher calories. Sugar is easy to spot on the food label as this is usually listed clearly.

As an example, when you research on Google regarding gluten-free corn chips, the food content of a typical product is listed as follows: 12 chips (28 g) contain 0 g glucose, 7 g fat, 14 g carbohydrate, 4 g protein, 100 mg sodium and 250 mg of potassium. It also lists that the total calories are 140, of which fat contributed to it 60 calories. 78% of the 80 calories left (namely 62.4 calories) came from the carbohydrate (starch in corn) and 22% of the remaining calories were protein derived (this I had to calculate). As the stomach digests the corn chips within half an hour into sugar, you really have eaten 62.4 calories from sugar. The Internet tells you that 2.3 g of sugar from a sugar cube are the equivalent of 9 calories. Our "sugar math" can be completed by doing this: 62.4 / 9 x 2.3 g = 15.94 or 16 grams of sugar. So, the food industry actually lied to you by saying that there was 0 g sugar in the 12 corn chips. What happened is that your body digested the 14 grams of carbs and converted it into sugar, which was absorbed into your blood stream. Your pancreas could tell you a story, because it had to produce some more insulin to keep your blood sugar level in balance!

I stopped buying dark chocolate, even the 85% variety as they are selling me 10 grams of sugar in a 40-gram helping (25% of sugar). All the health benefits are no longer applicable when you consume that much sugar with a supposedly healthy food item. So add up the sugar you are getting and add up the calories you are seeing listed. Usually, if the sugar content is high, the calories are high as well. So, here I am, drooling in front of a shelf with dark chocolate, yet I do not want the sugar that comes with the product. I don't subscribe to the theory that "a little bit does not harm". After too many "little bits" this statement loses ground. Maybe I'm a purist, but I still like that piece of chocolate with a tiny bit of sweetness. You may wonder how I solved the dark chocolate problem, which by the way would double as a gluten-free food: You buy 100 % unsweetened Baker's or other unsweetened chocolate (0 g sugar on the label) and liquefy it in a little bowl in a pot with hot water. Add a tiny bit of stevia sweetener and add a tiny bit of pure vanilla extract into the well-stirred chocolate liquid. Pour the content carefully into a square glass dish (watch it, hot!) and let it sit to cool down. When it is at room temperature, cut into smaller pieces, which you keep in a glass jar. This is 100% gluten-free, 100% chocolate, 0 % sugar and 100% healthy.

Conclusion

Not all is well in the gluten grocery row of your friendly super market. There are problems in that 20 to 25% of people believe they may have gluten sensitivity when in reality only 1% has this problem. The majority of people have not done a gluten-screening test, which would confirm that they have indeed celiac disease. As pointed out above, it is much more likely that a food sensitivity may be caused by another offending agent rather than gluten (milk sugar, fructose and sorbitol). Avoiding the offending food components is the treatment protocol.

Those who take in processed gluten-free food – all the cookies, crackers, cereals and breads - will expose themselves to unnecessary toxins and to extra sugar leading to obesity and metabolic syndrome that cause premature heart attacks and strokes. For those who do need to be on a strict gluten-free diet, they can safely do so by following a strict gluten free diet at home (preparing your own meals from healthy ingredients), preferably with organic foods. There are many websites that you can find online that have meal suggestions.

Sugar and Starch age you faster

Fareed Zacharia interviewed Chief Medical Correspondent Sanjay Gupta on CNN on Sept. 10, 2014 regarding why sugar is worse than fat.

I like to explain why it is important to rethink the issues of fat, cholesterol, sugar, starchy foods, longevity, prevention of cardiovascular diseases, strokes, heart attacks) and cancer.

I have written about this many times before, but perhaps an overview regarding these issues would be in order.

The Framingham Heart Study indicated first that too much cholesterol in our system was a problem leading to heart attacks and strokes. I reviewed this in my book published in 2014. As more research was done, the reasons for this have become clearer.

1.Liver metabolism

The liver plays a major role in the metabolism of glucose. Digestion of refined starchy foods starts in the mouth where amylase from the saliva digests the surface of the pasta or white bread you eat. The stomach carries on with this process and the job is finished in the small intestine with the help of pancreatic enzymes. This digestive process is so efficient that within 20 to 30 minutes all of the refined carbs from pasta, donuts and bread appear as sugar in the blood stream. The portal vein system that collects the nutrients from the gut delivers all sugar straight to the liver where it is reassembled into glucagon as the storage form in the liver and skeletal muscles. This would all be good, would we have periods of fasting in between our sugar consumption. Periods of famine are no longer part of modern civilization. It is no longer about feast or famine, but living in a world of consumerism. Most of the processed foods contain sugar and this leads to excess sugar uptake, which has to be processed by our liver. The end result is production of LDL cholesterol, oxidization of LDL cholesterol by sugar and in the process the production of VLDL (=very low-density lipoproteins) that leads directly to deposits in the arterial walls and to clogging of arteries. Triglycerides are also produced and deposited as fats (the cause of the obesity wave that we see around the industrial world).

2. Where does the fat that we see around us come from?

In the past we thought that consumption of too much saturated fat and cholesterol would be the cause for the accumulation of fat and cholesterol in the body. Now we know that this was an over-simplification. In fact more cholesterol and fat comes from metabolized sugar and with a slight time delay also from starchy foods.

Your liver metabolizes sugar and starchy foods (like pasta, white rice, white bread, potatoes, grapes, honey etc.) into LDL cholesterol, triglycerides, and fat. You still need to pay attention to the total fat content and the quality of fats you eat.

3. The finer points about subfractions of cholesterol

You have heard many times about the good (HDL) and the bad (LDL) cholesterol. Sugar and refined starches do not only lead to the production of LDL cholesterol, but also to oxidized LDL cholesterol, which is very aggressive (VLDL=very low-density lipoproteins) leading directly to deposits in the arterial walls and to clogging of arteries. Your doctor can order a detailed lipid profile test, if you belong into a higher risk group to determine your VLDL level.

It may surprise you to read that many of the foods that were demonized in the past 2 to 3 decades like whole eggs, unprocessed grass-fed red meat, coconut oil etc. are now seen as being beneficial for you.

But there are provisos: check that you have enough molecularly distilled omega-3 fatty acids, enough vitamin D3, vitamin K2 and calcium in your diet or supplement with these. This will make sure that calcium will leave the blood stream and not lead to arteriosclerosis, the medical term for hardening of arteries. This is particularly important for women in menopause for osteoporosis prevention. Vitamin K2 causes calcium to enter into the bones where calcium is needed for healthy bone structure. The anti-inflammatory effect of vitamin D3 and of the omega-3 fatty acids will prevent arthritis, strokes, heart attacks and cancer. Both vitamin D3 and vitamin K2 help to get calcium into the bone: calcium is better absorbed in the gut in the presence of vitamin D3, vitamin K2 removes calcium from the blood circulation by having calcium incorporated into bone; this last step is also helped by vitamin D3.

4. Four major conditions causing heart attacks and strokes

Williams Textbook of Endocrinology explains that only 4 conditions have been proven over the years to lead to serious hardening of arteries causing strokes and heart attacks: dyslipidemia (high triglycerides, high LDL cholesterol and VLDL), hypertension, cigarette smoking, and/or diabetes. What has not been appreciated until recently is the fact that sugar and refined starchy foods metabolized by the liver are the culprits in causing plaque in arteries as the oxidized LDL cholesterol is aggressively invading the arterial wall and it is also inflammatory. A total cholesterol level greater than 5.2 mmol/L (200 mg/dL) has been shown to be associated with increased heart attacks and strokes. Dietary changes, days of fasting and weight loss have all been shown to stabilize and reduce plaque lesions and reduce heart attacks and strokes. It is the rupture of unstable plaques that leads to attraction of platelets and thrombus formation. It is this localized thrombosis that leads to the closure of coronary arteries or brain vessels causing heart attacks and strokes. Williams Textbook of Endocrinology states that there are 9 factors that determine whether we get a stroke or heart attack, the four factors mentioned above (dyslipidemia, hypertension, cigarette smoking, diabetes) and abdominal obesity, lack of physical activity, low daily fruit and vegetable consumption, alcohol overconsumption, and a psychosocial risk. This latter factor includes any kind of chronic stress like interpersonal stress at work or home, depression, financial stress, major life events like marriage, death, divorce, and lack of control. Counseling is useful for support regarding psychosocial risk factors. It is significant to note that several studies have shown that paying attention to these 9 risk factors can prevent 90% of heart attacks and strokes. Managing stress effectively helps. We can use relaxation techniques, prayer or meditation to seek quietness and calm our minds. But there are also difficult life circumstances that can overwhelm us. In these situations we should not be shy to seek professional help. Recognizing the stressors in our lives and managing stress as well as avoiding the physical health risks will contribute to good overall health.

Conclusion

Where does this leave us? For decades we have been told that saturated fats and cholesterol in our diet were the culprits and we replaced them with sugar that is part of a low-fat diet. We need to pay attention to the glycemic index and cut out high glycemic foods as discussed in the prior section "carbs". However, it is OK to eat some carbs from the medium glycemic food list and most of our carbs from the low glycemic food list. With regard to fat it is important to consume only the healthy fats including omega-3 fatty acids. Olive oil has several healthy ingredients in it that lower LDL cholesterol and increases the protective HDL cholesterol. By taking care of the 4 major causes of heart

attacks and strokes and also attending to the additional minor contributors mentioned above you will be able to eliminate 90% of the cardiovascular events. As you change these things you will also prevent many cancers: you changed the body metabolism, avoided chronic inflammation and this is known to prevents cancer as well. Finally, pay attention to stress management. Body and mind work together.

Healthy sugar substitutes

It is true that sweets are not good for you because they lead to fat accumulation and to diabetes. I explain how this works below. But who says you cannot sweeten your life with healthy ingredients? Not all sugar substitutes are the same; some are awful, some are in between and one is good (see below).

General information why sweets and starches are bad for you

There is a triple whammy from sweets that you don't really want

a) First, sugar gets absorbed really fast through the gut wall and arrives in your blood stream within 15 to 20 minutes. Starches can be just as powerful in terms of blood sugar surges, but it takes perhaps 30 to 40 minutes for the peak of blood sugar to occur. The end result is the same: whether you load up with a pizza, a doughnut or a sugar-loaded soda drink, your pancreas reacts the same way. It produces a lot of extra insulin to bring the blood sugar level down. When you do this day after day, your pancreas gets used to overproducing insulin and you develop insulin resistance meaning that your insulin receptors that are on

every cell surface get tired and become less sensitive to insulin. Due to insulin resistance the muscle cells and the liver cells do not take up sugar (in the form of glucose) as easily as before.

b) Second, excess sugar cannot be stored as glycogen (the storage form of glucose in the liver and the muscles), so the liver converts excess glucose into triglycerides. White blood cells called macrophages take up oxidized fatty acids. These attach to the inner lining of the arteries and lead to atheromatous plaques, the first stage of hardening of the arteries.

c) Third, glucose is an oxidizing agent that will oxidize LDL cholesterol. This makes the LDL particles much denser and forms the so-called very dense LDL lipoprotein fraction (VDLDL) that can be detected in special blood tests.

Not surprisingly people who consume sugar, sweets, soft drinks and starches on a regular basis will have very dense LDL particles (=VDLDL, also called "pattern B-LDL"). The treatment for this is to quit sugar and starchy foods.

You can read more detail about how sugar from a high carb/low fat diet makes you sick in a blog (see under references).

The food industry's answer to low carb diet drinks and low sugar foods

Many years back the food industry decided to offer alternative diet drinks that would not contain sugar, but instead have aspartame in it.

Dr. Blaylock has researched excitotoxins like MSG and aspartame (NutraSweet) and urges you to abandon both. I agree with him. But while we are discussing this,

don't take other artificial sweeteners like sodium cyclamate in Canada (Sweet'N Low). Are you thinking of taking sucralose (Splenda) instead? Think again. What the industry seems to have forgotten is that it was originally developed as an insecticide. This website states "Sucralose was actually discovered while trying to create a new insecticide". A researcher tasted it and found it exceedingly sweet. I have done the experiment myself in Hawaii where small ants are ubiquitous. I took a package of Splenda from a coffee shop and sprinkled it on an ant trail. It was interesting for me to watch: in the beginning the ants were reluctant to eat it, but after a few hours they came and took it in. One day later there were only shriveled up dead ants left in the area where Splenda had been sprinkled. Proof enough for me that Splenda was developed as an insecticide! Did I still consider it as a sweetener? Of course not! I believe that insecticides, no matter how sweet they are, are not suitable for human consumption.

In the Splenda marketing scheme it was first decided to introduce Splenda gradually into diabetic foods as a sweetener, then later sell it to the public at large. Don't fall for it. Even though it is still labeled as "harmless", there are already enough reports that persons using it have experienced gastric reflux (GERD). We should also remember that it was a side product of insecticide research, and insecticides have the undesirable quality of being xenoestrogens, which block estrogen receptors in women. As a result of that estrogen can no longer access the body cells, including the heart. The final consequence for a woman is a higher risk for cardio-vascular disease. This can cause heart attacks, strokes and cancer. In men estrogen-blocking xenoestrogens can cause breast growth and erectile dysfunction.

The natural sweeteners

One wonders why the food industry did not choose healthy sweeteners like stevia that has been used for decades in Japan and hundreds of years in South America.

Other sweeteners like xylitol, sorbitol, maltitol, mannitol, glycerol, and lactitol are sugar alcohols. In higher dosages they lead to stomach cramps and loose bowels. Contrary to what many believe they have calories, but much less than sugar, so they are perceived as "safe" as a dietary supplement for weight loss. These alcoholic sugar compounds still produce partial LDL oxidization, interfere with weight loss and still lead to a certain insulin response. Stevia, a natural sweetener from the leave of a South American plant is safer and without any calories.

The key is that stevia will not oxidize your LDL cholesterol and will not cause a hyper-insulin response following a meal. It is metabolically neutral. It is the ideal sweetener for people who want to avoid the additional insulin surge and desire to lose some weight. It is also safe as it is no excitotoxin. The FDA has recognized stevia as "generally recognized as safe" (GRAS) in 2008.

What about fructose, agave syrup, honey, brown rice malt syrup, fruit juice concentrates, refined fructose, and maple syrup?

The problem is that they are all sugars, which cause a full insulin response leading to obesity, diabetes and hardening of the arteries. This causes heart attacks and strokes. These natural sugar products also oxidize LDL cholesterol, which initiates plaque formation as discussed above; this is the first step leading to hardening of the arteries. It took the medical profession 30 years of observing that a low fat/ high carb diet makes us fat and causes heart attacks, leads to strokes and causes diabetes. Let's not make the mistake of trusting the food industry and mindlessly swallow so-called natural other sugars and sugar substitutes like xylitol, sorbitol, maltitol, mannitol, glycerol, and lactitol. You may want to chew the odd gum with xylitol, as this will prevent cavities in your teeth. But otherwise it is much safer to just stick to Stevia to sweeten your tea, coffee or food. Stevia has to be used in very small amounts, as too much of it can leave you with a spiky, slightly bitter taste. Some brands tend to have this more than others. I'm not running commercials for companies, but I found from my own observations that products like stevia from New Roots in Canada and stevia from KAL in the US are good products with no bitter after taste. You have to try out, which one is your favorite.

Conclusion

Sugar is an emotional topic that can get people caught up in heated discussions. The sugar industry and the sugar substitute industry have also powerful lobby groups that provide the internet and the popular press with conflicting stories to convince you to buy their product. This section was meant as a no-nonsense guide to get you removed from the high-risk group of candidates for heart attacks, strokes or diabetes. Let's not forget the metabolism behind the various sugars and starchy foods described above, which I have explained in more detail in my book published in 2014. Forget the emotions of severing yourself from your favorite fix and stick to a tiny amount of stevia that can replace the familiar sweet taste that you have become accustomed to from childhood onward. At least this is what I do. The only alternative would be to take the plunge and cut out any sweet substance altogether, which I am not prepared to do. If you can do it, by all means go ahead.

A biased Soda study - sweet promises and a bitter truth

Recently the media reviewed an industry-sponsored study entitled: "Diet soda helps weight loss, industry-funded study finds". Before you get too excited about this study, let me tell you that you are being deceived. Essentially the study compared 150 overweight or obese people on water and a similar group of people on diet sodas. Both groups were counseled on the benefits of exercise and a healthier diet. At the end of 12 weeks the water group that did not drink diet sodas had lost 9 pounds, while the diet soda group that continued their former habit lost 13 pounds. The question now is why this 4 pound difference? The sponsor of the study would like you to think that the soda diet drink is healthier, because it helps you to lose weight. Let me explain to you that there are a few flaws in the study as follows.

***1. Most often there are confounding errors in industry-sponsored studies:* Even though it looks on the surface that the two groups were comparable, researchers should have checked out various parameters like sex distribution, other underlying illnesses, mental state (depressed or not etc.), diabetes and other factors to make sure that there is no metabolic bias between the two groups from the start of the study.**

***2. Deception is built into study:* We know from other studies that on the long-term diet sodas lead to weight gain by stimulating your appetite for sweets and their subsequent consumption. Often short-term studies show the opposite effect, so it would be false to assume that long-term results would be similar. But most readers who read this quickly would be tempted to think "so it must be**

OK to continue to consume diet soda drinks!" Off you go to the grocery store and buy another 6 or 12 pack. That's exactly what the industry-sponsored study set out to do. Somewhere in the back room of a big soft drink corporation the executives discussed among themselves that their sales statistics were bad; the sales of diet soft drinks were down; there was too much negative press fuelled by the health food industry. They had to do something about this, so they designed a study where the good guy was the diet soft drink. If the consumer is not buying the results, at least the study helped to confuse people and whenever there is confusion, at least part of the confused population will return to their old habits. After all the study showed "it is OK".

3. Excitotoxins are not OK: Unfortunately all artificial sweeteners are toxic to your brain, they are excitotoxins. MSG is another excitotoxin. The only exception is the natural sweetener stevia, a plant product, which is OK. Splenda is an insecticide, so this belongs to the xenoestrogens, bad for you as it acts like a foreign estrogen and has cancer-promoting qualities when exposed to it for several decades. The rest of the artificial sweeteners are excitotoxins: they burn your brain cells very slowly and can lead to dementia. Unfortunately they are addicting and your brain will make you feel good when you drink more of it. So, the real reason why the study group on diet sodas did better than the water group is because they did not have to change that habit, there was no withdrawal to deal with, and they felt fine. So they could concentrate on dieting and exercising and of course you would lose 13 pounds in 12 weeks doing that. The water group on the other hand had to cope with diet soda withdrawal and on top was challenged by an exercise and weight loss program. As there was no diet restriction, they could compensate a bit for their trouble of withdrawal

and eat a few muffins or some extra bread to make up for the lack of their comfort diet drink fix (the satisfaction of consuming the excitotoxin). This slick, short-term study design is what should have alarmed the publisher to ask a few hard questions.

4. There needs to be an internal logic in the study: **Let's do a thought experiment where we repeat the study and start with two comparable overweight/obese groups of people and put them on no sugar and no refined carbs for 2 weeks and also on no diet sodas for the same time. After two weeks they are both accustomed to this diet and the no diet soda habit and they have probably lost the same amount of weight from the calorie restriction. Now we start the one group on diet sodas and the other group on water, but strictly controlled for a similar calorie intake in terms of other foods or drinks as much as is humanly possible. I would predict that after 12 weeks the water group will have at least lost the same weight as the diet soda group, if not more. The diet soda group likely will have had some problems with sugar craving and may have had more dietary indiscretions (sneaking in snacks and underreporting them), but this would show up as weight gain.**

You may be proud of having completed this well controlled study. The trouble is that your industry sponsor that produces the diet drinks will not like this outcome and would not allow the results to be published. In fact that kind of result would be actively suppressed.

Conclusion

The diet soda study discussed here is a lesson in biased publishing. We are constantly bombarded by an endless string of meaningless publications that are designed to make the consumer insecure, or bias us for accepting a

company's product in the hope of achieving a certain result, like high sales. Even, if this is not accomplished the company has sold enough of their product just for giving it a try. Beware of the door-to-door sales person. This figure is very much present right in this publication. In this case it is the sales pitch of the diet soda manufacturers! You are looking at a study that was designed to make you buy more of the excitotoxin (aspartame or other artificial sweeteners), which likely contributed to your extra weight or obesity in the first place. It's up to you to shut the door on this sales pitch. Instead of a diet soda I suggest you make your own drink: squeeze half an organic lemon and top this with mineral water of your choice. Sweeten it with a tiny amount of stevia. This has no calories and does not stimulate you to eat more sugar and starchy foods; this drink quenches any thirst and you even get some water-soluble vitamins in the process.

Avoid restaurants or find an organic one

Recently I saw a flyer of a fast food chain restaurant entitled "Food Fact". Interestingly you get the contents of a list of bakery items, warm breakfast items, burgers, sandwiches and wraps for lunch as well as yogurt parfaits and fruit cups.

I have to commend the restaurant chain to attempt to educate their customers by listing the content of each item. They have listed the serving size broken down into calories, total fat, saturated fat, trans fat, cholesterol, sugar, protein, dietary fiber, vitamin C, A, calcium and iron.

Based on my dietary habits I need to check this list.

No trans fat

Years ago I have given up on trans fats because trans fat contain free radicals that accelerate hardening of the arteries. Granted, the percentage is low, but 20% come from natural meats and 80% from processed foods. It is the 80% from processed foods that I avoid. I reviewed the CDC website that answers the question “what is fat” (see references). This eliminates the baked sweet pieces like croissants, cookies, raisin bran muffins, oat fudge bars and even spinach feta wraps.

Total fat

Now we come to total fat. The content list shows me that calories in total and fat content in total are closely related. But you reach the peak when you swallowed a sausage, egg and cheddar breakfast sandwich. These alone account for 500 calories. This is also high in cholesterol and high in sodium, so not really on my list of desirable foods.

Sodium content

I am now getting concerned about my blood pressure as I follow the sodium content. Who would have thought that a spinach feta wrap has more than 800mg of sodium? And ham and a Swiss Panini have more than 1500 mg of sodium? Literally 50% of the food list would not be on my menu, if I want to limit my sodium intake to 400mg or less per helping. Especially the sandwiches are out!

Hidden sugar

So, now I am looking at yoghurt for a light snack, but suddenly the sugar column has sprung up from 1-2 mg of sugar content in simple sandwiches to 37 to 55 mg of sugar for a honey creek yoghurt parfait or a strawberry blueberry parfait. It is not the yoghurt, it’s not the fruit, it is extra sugar, and honey or high-fructose corn syrup mixed in here. This is definitely not what I am going to choose.

Refined carbs

Although the carbs by weight do not appear too high on the list, it is the total of sugar and carbs and the fat that has been added, which add up very quickly to hefty calorie sums in all of the foods. I am shaking my head and I absolutely cannot find anything that is healthy and would merit a further look.

Missing greens

I am missing vegetables and salads. The only thing I see that I can eat is their classic oatmeal, which has 160 calories with a nut medley topping. I may add a decaf-coffee sweetened with my own stevia that I brought along and some cream (because that's how I still like it, having been raised in Germany). If I have my decaf-coffee, I better skip the classical oatmeal, because I am sure the oatmeal is not organic, which translates into exposure to herbicides like glyphosate.

Homemade food

So I had no luck at this establishment. As a result I'll go over to the health food store and to the grocery store and load up on organic foods, meat, lettuce, broccoli, peppers, spinach, organic olive oil and balsamic vinegar. And yes, I'll get a tub of plain goat or organic yogurt. Organic walnut halves are also on the list (quite expensive, I must say).

I suddenly realize that now I have all of the ingredients to be independent from a restaurant. I can prepare my own food, and I can do it the way I want it, not how the food industry wants me to eat it.

If I ate the food industry's way, the salt content would send my blood pressure through the roof and I would get hardening of the arteries within the shortest time (from refined sugar, starchy foods and trans fats).

I find the taste of home cooked meals superb. All of the flavors are there. Of course, I do not mind spending the extra money on the organic food, because the tastes are the way my grandmother's food used to taste. I rarely add salt and my blood pressure is 105/65; so something must be going right.

I am thinking what would happen, if more people would do what I do: avoid restaurants, especially fast food places, pack your own lunch box with an organic salad and enjoy dinner at home. It can be simple, tasty, healthy, and economical. Nobody needs to be an accomplished chef to do that. Would there be pressure on the food industry to open up organic restaurants and offer alternatives to those who want to enjoy healthy, tasty foods? Or are the fast food places here to stay forever and ever? It will be consumer habits that make that decision.

Conclusion

In this section I just took you to one of those fast food places that actually list their food content. Listing it does not really help when the whole list consists almost exclusively of foods that are having serious drawbacks, be it in the addition of too much sodium, fats, sugar or refined carbs.

You do not want to get accelerated hardening of your arteries from too much fat, trans fat, sugar and starchy foods. You don't want to get high blood pressure from too much salt day after day. You may want to rethink that processed foods are really lacking the nutrition that your body needs to function well and stay healthy. A lot of the processed food are best to be thrown out. You need fresh, organic vegetables and green leafed vegetables like lettuce, spinach, Swiss chard and others. Maybe you want a vegetable omelet for breakfast with egg white, spinach, peppers and Swiss chard? Take charge of your own life. Look after your own affairs. This includes what you do in your kitchen and what foods you consume.

Probiotics, an old fact newly discovered

Growing up in Germany after the Second World War I remember that every so often newspaper headings showed an older person in the nineties when the average life expectancy was in the late 60's. The reporter asked, "What did you do to turn that old?" The answer was often that the person ate a lot of yogurt.

This did not sink into mainstream medicine at that time, and people did not really believe this statement. How could eating yogurt make a person live longer?

Fast forward to 2015. You read about probiotics in magazines, on the Internet, and get exposed to it in TV commercials.

In the Wikipedia it is accepted that yogurt can help seniors who have a lower bifidus bacteria population in their colon to rebalance their gut flora, which will prevent colon cancer. It also describes that yeast infections in women can be helped by yogurt.

In the meantime probiotics have been developed and concentrations like 20 to 80 billion bacteria per capsule with a mix of Lactobacillus and Bifidobacterium species are available in the health food store for prevention.

The medical profession has studied the effects of higher potency probiotics and came to the conclusion that probiotics have indeed effects on the body far beyond the gut.

Here are a few highlights.

Bowel disease improves

In cases of bacterial or viral diarrhea the frequency of bowel movements and the intensity of bowel cramps gets helped within a few days, and recovery from the diarrhea is much faster with a probiotic than without the use of it. Patient with irritable bowel syndrome and ulcerative colitis are helped with probiotics. Both constipation and diarrhea in otherwise healthy people are helped as well.

Immune system booster

The small bowel has been known for a long time to have clusters of immune cells within the bowel wall. Together they are a formidable immune organ in the gut, which connects to the blood and the rest of the immune system throughout the body (lymph glands, spleen, bone marrow). Specifically it has been proven in humans that macrophages, natural killer (NK) cells and cytotoxic T-lymphocytes, which are the workhorses of the immune system, are all stimulated by probiotics.

Less respiratory infections

School children were given 1 capsule of probiotics twice per day for 3 months and flu symptoms and absenteeism were observed due to colds and flus. When they did get a viral infection, the illness had a shorter course, resulting in much less school absenteeism over the course of the trial when compared to a placebo group. It seems that a healthy gut flora stimulates the immune system to work at its best.

Cancer prevention

To a certain degree cancer can be prevented by probiotics and other nutritional factors. Breast cancer is one of the cancers where probiotics have been shown to be effective in reducing disease.

Apparently the probiotic bacteria bind to the cancer causing factors (carcinogens) that some of the bad gut bacteria produce. Probiotics also suppress other bacteria that convert pro-carcinogens into carcinogens. This is not all: the probiotics also interfere with enzymes involved in the production of carcinogens in the gut, which stimulates the gut immune cells to produce cytokines that are needed in the battle against early cancer. Probiotics play a role in multiple processes that help the body to fight cancer, not only in the gut, but also in the rest of the body!

Probiotics help diabetes get better

How can gut bacteria help diabetes, which is an endocrinological disease? Both human and animal studies have shown that insulin resistance is improved by probiotics. In a 6-week study both blood sugar levels and hemoglobin A1C values (that measure long-term control of diabetes) dropped significantly by eating 300 grams of yoghurt per day when compared to a control group who did not.

Obesity

Probiotics given to mothers at least one month prior to birth and at least up to 6 months after birth prevented excessive weight gain in both the mothers and their children. A lot of the inflammatory substances associated with obesity are suppressed by probiotics.

Probiotics reduce cardiovascular risk

Several studies have shown that probiotics lower LDL cholesterol, total cholesterol and inflammatory markers in the blood stream resulting in lower risk for hardening of the arteries.

One should not look at probiotics as a single factor for prevention of heart attacks and strokes, but combine probiotics with exercise and a diet that is low in refined carbs. High sugar and starch diets lead to absorption of sugar in the stomach and small intestine. This results in a lack of nutrients to support the gut flora. When probiotics are combined with vegetables and lettuce there is the proper mix of fiber, minerals and other nutrients to sustain balanced bacteria in the bowels for preventing heart attacks and strokes and keeping inflammatory markers down. The combination of organic food (to avoid antibiotic residues in our diet), fruit and vegetables combined with probiotics will protect you from heart attacks and strokes.

Conclusion

Maybe the newspaper articles in Germany after the Second World War were right that something in yogurt (Lactobacillus and Bifidobacterium species) could make you live longer. The explanation seems simple: add probiotics to your diet and you will have a better immune system, get less respiratory infections, prevent heart attacks and strokes and prevent obesity and cancer. All of this in combination will lead to healthier lives, and more people will live to tell about it.

Olive oil

As the Mediterranean diet includes cooking with olive oil, I thought that a review of what olive oil does is in order. In the past the medical profession believed that the monounsaturated fatty acids in olive oil would be the reason why olive oil is protective of the heart. However, newer studies have shown that it is the polyphenols and among these in particular hydroxytyrosol that lower blood pressure and protect you from hardening of the arteries.

In a 2012 study from Spain it was found that mortality from heart attacks was 44% lower than that of a control group who did not incorporate olive oil in their diet.

How polyphenols in olive oil work for you

Only a minimum of two tablespoons of extra virgin olive oil per day protects you from heart disease. It does so by reducing the total cholesterol level in the blood as well as the LDL cholesterol level. At the same time the more polyphenol is contained in olive oil (such as in extra virgin olive oil), the more HDL your body will produce, which is essential to extract oxidized LDL from arterial plaque. On top of that polyphenol rich olive oil will increase the size of the HDL particles (these larger particles are called HDL2), which are more efficient in extracting oxidized LDL from arterial plaques. A Sept. 2014 study in humans showed that higher polyphenol olive oil as found in extra virgin olive oil caused an increase in the more effective HDL2 particles. This cleans out plaques from arteries more efficiently than the regular, cheaper olive oil.

Endothelial function

The endothelium is the lining of the arteries. Normal endothelial functioning involves widening of the arteries and maintaining flexibility. The body achieves this through production of a signal molecule, called nitric oxide; the endothelial cells that line our arteries from inside produce it. Exercise increases the production of nitric oxide as well.

In a group of patients with poor endothelial function 2 tablespoons of olive oil (polyphenol rich) per day given over 4 months (the time of the study) showed a significant improvement of endothelial function.

The authors suggested that an enzyme in the endothelial cells, called nitric oxide synthase is being stimulated by components of polyphenol-rich olive oil. This leads to protracted release of nitric oxide, which in turn keeps blood vessels flexible and wide open. Other investigators found that olive oil can influence even a hereditary gene variant of endothelial nitric oxide synthase found in people with a history of premature heart attacks and metabolic syndrome. This high-risk group of people should take extra virgin olive oil regularly to prevent premature heart attacks and strokes.

Endothelial dysfunction occurs when the arteries no longer can deliver adequate amounts of blood to vital organs like the heart or the brain. Endothelial dysfunction is present in patients with type 2 diabetes, obesity, high blood pressure and metabolic syndrome. Introducing extra virgin olive oil in the diet of these patients will help restore their endothelial function.

Lowering blood pressure

In a study on 23 hypertensive patients it was shown as far back as in 2000 that extra virgin olive oil over 6 months allowed physicians to reduce high blood pressure medications by 48%. When the study was crossed over, the reverse was the case for the control group on sunflower oil that had no such effect.

Based on what was said about endothelial function above, it is easy to understand that the polyphenols of olive oil released nitric oxide, which is known to lower blood pressure. This is an important finding as high blood pressure is a known risk factor for the development of hardening of the coronary arteries leading to heart attacks, to congestive heart failure, but also to strokes. Regular intake of 2 tablespoons of extra virgin olive oil often will reverse high blood pressure and restore normal endothelial function.

Preventing heart attacks and strokes

In April of 2013 The New England Journal of Medicine published a Spanish diet study that showed that participants on a Mediterranean diet with olive oil or nuts had 30% less heart attacks over 5 years than a control group on a low fat diet. Other studies have also shown that olive oil and omega-3 fatty acids play a big role in preventing heart attacks and strokes. We also know that regular exercise reduces the risk further; so does keeping your body mass index below 25.0. Extra virgin olive oil is part of the protection from heart attacks and strokes, but it did not show protection against cancer.

Conclusion

It is a simple fact that incorporating 2 tablespoons of virgin olive oil in your daily food intake will definitely have all of the beneficial effects described above. It is readily available, is inexpensive and very effective. It is also not difficult to work into your eating routine: add olive oil and vinegar or lemon juice to your salads, and cook with olive oil. If you have not totaled 30 grams (2 tablespoons), then make up the difference by eating an extra teaspoon full of olive oil. This is not all! You need to cut down on processed foods as they are made with the wrong oils, such as safflower

oil, corn oil, soybean oil and others. These are omega-6 containing oils that cause heart attacks and strokes. They are cheap oils used by food processors, and they are not doing anything for your health!

I would suggest that you read more about the powerful role of prevention that extra virgin olive oil has in our diet. Buy it and stick to it as a new healthy lifestyle habit. Two tablespoons a day is the weapon against cardiovascular disease!

Pure water

Water has been in the news a lot: there has been the Toledo, Ohio incident affecting 400,000 residents because toxins of algae from Lake Erie entered into the public water system. At about the same time in northern British Columbia, Canada there was a broken dam from a mining company's toxic wastewater reservoir spilling toxic wastewater into the Fraser River drinking water system.

Between 60 and 70% of our bodies are made up of water. We need water for a multitude of biochemical reactions that constantly take place within us. We need water to "run the engine". This includes detoxification of our bodies as water is a large part of our kidney excretions (urine) and our stools still have a significant percentage of water. Water is also the basis for our blood circulation.

Knowing this, it is important that we insist on drinking only pure water. In the following I will describe why this can be a problem and how to solve this problem.

Brief history of water purification

A private company developed the first sand filter for water purification in Scotland in 1804.

Based on this success, the Chelsea Waterworks Company in London was founded in 1829, which was the first

public water supply in the world. When a cholera epidemic hit London in 1854, physician Dr. Snow discovered that cholera was confined to those districts in London where water was not purified, and he provided the authorities with a dot map depicting the cholera cases in London, which correlated with the water system that used no filtration methods. When the pumps were switched off in this district of London, the cholera epidemic subsided.

Europe adopted the English model in the late 1800's and added sewage treatment plants in order to separate wastewater from drinking water. The first sewage treatment plant was built in Frankfurt, Germany in 1887. This was necessary because of huge epidemics of cholera and typhoid fever that swept through Europe. When separation of sewage and drinking water was achieved, these epidemics stopped.

It is interesting that minimal water standards were introduced in the US only in 1914, and it took until 1940 before water purity was legislated federally.

Toxins in water

Townships have to get the drinking water they pipe into your house from somewhere. Often this is a lake, an artesian well or several artesian wells combined; in the past it was from rivers, but they are now mostly contaminated with sewage and chemicals. The latest example is Flint, Michigan where lead poisoning occured on a large scale. Lead from the polluted Flint River entered the public water system and made international headlines in January of 2016. We like to think that in our times of regulated water safety such disasters would not happy any more, but they do!

There is the added problem that natural soil compositions vary tremendously throughout a country. One example is arsenic that is contained naturally in soils of some areas in the world, so-called "hot spots", and the drinking water can be high in arsenic in those places.

It follows from here that some springs can also be contaminated with arsenic and other heavy metals. Heavy metals poison our internal enzyme systems and interfere with the body's metabolism.

A well is more likely to contain arsenic than a river or lake as a water source. But we do not only concern ourselves with toxins; viruses and bacteria are also a problem that can cause water related diseases.

Bacterial and viral contamination

In Europe, before cities built sewage systems, it was not uncommon that excrements from humans and animals found their way into the well that was used for drinking water. We like to think that we are safe now with all of the laws and measures in place, but the various news stories teach us otherwise. Common bacterial contaminants are Salmonella, E.coli (strain O157:H7), Giardia lamblia, Legionella, the parasite Cryptosporidium and others.

In Canada there was a tragic incident in 2000 where thousands of residents of Walkerton, a small town in Ontario were exposed to E.coli (strain O157:H7). This was due to a malfunctioning chlorination unit, but those who were responsible for water quality maintenance were denying it and were not even properly trained to run the chlorination equipment.

Water testing

Water testing is at the beginning of any water purification system and intermittent ongoing testing is at the center of monitoring water quality on a permanent basis. Water inspectors need to constantly monitor the water source, the water purification process and the delivery system.

Many people in rural Canadian or US towns depend on well water. The same logic of monitoring water quality applies for well water as it does for municipal water; but well water monitoring is on a smaller scale.

You want to know what your water is like. It is not difficult to find out: take a water sample and have it analyzed by a water company. Depending on the results the water company will advise you what kind of filter you will need.

The first purification stage typically is an activated carbon filter that removes organic compounds, radon and other impurities. Every three or four days the filter automatically backwashes and cleans itself for about 45 minutes. Once a year or with good water quality up to every three years the activated carbon has to be removed and replaced by a new filter. This type of filter is also useful for people who are on municipal water, but want to remove the halogens (fluoride, bromide, chloride) used to disinfect municipal water.

The second stage is an ultraviolet irradiation device. This disinfects the water from any bacteria, viruses or parasites just prior to coming to your water tap.

It is recommended that you also install a reverse osmosis system under your main kitchen sink. It will provide you with purified drinking water. Water produced by this filter goes through additional activated carbon filters and finally must pass through a porous membrane where only water can pass through, but heavy metals and other impurities will not. During an outbreak of Cryptosporidium in 1996 in Kelowna, BC those who had a reverse osmosis system were safe from this pathogen.

You can brush your teeth with confidence with reverse osmosis water, even if your tap water is contaminated.

Proper water purification

If you are on municipal water, find out what water purification system the municipality is using to ensure water safety. Usually there is a first step of a slow sand filter, where the raw water is first purified, then it undergoes a water chlorination, bromination or fluoridation process, which is done to remove bacteria and viruses. We know, however from a series of outbreaks of Cryptosporidium gastroenteritis cases in municipalities that only used this two-stage purification process that this was inadequate. It was that a third step, namely ultraviolet germicidal irradiation, which was missing to eradicate this microscopic parasite.

Cryptosporidium was the problem behind a drinking water problem in the summer of 1996 in Kelowna, BC, the town of the interior of BC, Canada where I live. 50,000 residents had to get their drinking water from water trucks that were parked at certain locations of the town (about 40% of the population was affected by this water problem). Following this disaster Kelowna now has a modern ultraviolet irradiation system in place as a third water purification step.

Immune system compromised people

People whose immune system is compromised such as AIDS patients or patients who had chemotherapy for cancer are very susceptible to Cryptosporidium and other parasites, bacteria and viruses. For them it is particularly important that the third stage, the ultraviolet irradiation step be part of the municipal water treatment process. If this is missing, have a home unit installed by a water company.

Some people may shy away from the cost of the installation of a purification unit. Clean drinking water remains important. Another avenue is purchasing purified water for cooking and drinking in large bottles from a water company.

Conclusion

It is interesting to see how in Europe the history of water purification has been tightly linked to the history of cholera and typhoid fever epidemics; the quest for learning from these mistakes of the past has brought new solutions. In the past the mistake had been that wastewater contaminated the drinking water sources. To our modern thinking this seems unimaginable. But recent events that we read about in the news remind us that we cannot be lax on water safety and purification. It is a reality that the same mistakes from the past are still sporadically made now! Know your water source; know the water quality of the water you brush your teeth with (for instance use only bottled water for this in Mexico). Remember that in many development countries, to which you may travel, there is no clear separation of drinking water and wastewater and there may not be a three-phase filtration system in place that I described above.

Enjoy drinking your clean, refreshing water!

Food safety

Although food safety is always important, it is particularly important in summer. With tropical storm Arthur (July 2014) and others there were many power failures and much spoiled food due to non-functioning refrigerators had to be discarded.

Take a summer garden party as an example: food is outside in warmer temperatures, and it does not take long before salmonella or enteric bacteria multiply in mayonnaise, which acts like a growth medium. Traveler's diarrhea is common in development countries. Bugs such as Shigella, enterotoxigenic E. coli, Campylobacter jejuni, Salmonella species and others are the most common bacteria that cause food poisoning. A bunch of others have interesting sounding names but are ugly dinner companions: the rotavirus subtypes and the parasites Entamoeba histolytica, Giardia lamblia, Cryptosporidium species and Cyclospora cayetanensis are also frequent offenders that make people sick, make them vomit or cause diarrhea.

How is food poisoning caused?

Causes of food poisoning vary from food to food and between developed countries to developing countries. Bacterial contamination of meats or poultry is particularly common, and prompt refrigeration at 4 degrees Celsius or lower (38 F or lower) is important to prevent bacteria from multiplying to prevent food poisoning. People with contaminated hands that handle food in the retail grocery business can introduce bacteria or noroviruses into the food chain. Cross contamination by cutting meat on a cutting board and subsequently cutting lettuce for a salad that is uncooked is a common source of food poisoning. While the bacteria or viruses of the meat that was cut and subsequently cooked is now safe to eat, the salad with the bacteria or viruses from the uncooked meat is causing food poisoning. 75% of oysters harvested around the shelves in Great Britain are contaminated with norovirus. It is important therefore to boil the oysters well to inactivate the norovirus; half-cooked or raw oysters are simply not acceptable.

Pay attention to food preparation

Before you prepare a meal, make sure that all of the ingredients that come from packages have an expiry date well beyond the date when you prepare the meal. Anything that is beyond the expiry date may have a larger number of bacteria or viruses in them that could transfer into the rest of the meal.

Keep in mind that during the summer outside temperatures are well beyond room temperature, and it does not take long for bacteria to multiply at higher temperatures. The danger zone is between 40°F (4°C) and 140°F (60°C) where bacterial growth can occur. On many occasions scientists have measured that bacterial growth can double every 20 minutes, so within only one or two hours food such as mayonnaise, milk or eggs are spoiled!

Never leave barbecued meats lying around and only deep-freeze them later. When you thaw them in preparation for another meal in the future, you are dealing with spoiled food that already has bacteria in it as they grew before you have frozen the spoiled meat. Spoiled meat remains spoiled meat, even when you have stored it in the freezer! Throw it out.

Interrupt the infectious chain

The key in food preparation and cooking as well as in safe refrigeration storage is to interrupt the infectious chain. If you get meat from the store, cook it thoroughly so it is safe to eat. The cooking process will destroy bacteria.

Drink bottled or boiled water. Avoid ice cubes, as they may have been prepared with contaminated water. Avoid eating raw food. Eat salad only after it was thoroughly washed with clean water. In development countries or areas of questionable water supply go without salad until you enter a country where general hygienic standards are observed. Peel fruit yourself; don't eat fruit salads prepared by others. Generally speaking, food should be eaten hot. Avoid raw and poorly cooked seafood; invariably this is a risk for exposing yourself to unknown bacteria or viruses.

Eating in a restaurant is not as safe as eating at someone's home.

When you think about summer recreation, think about swimming pools; think also about recreational pools that may also be contaminated. If there is no appropriate chlorination equipment present, it is unsafe to use that pool.

Treatment of traveler's diarrhea

If you should get abdominal pain, diarrhea and vomiting you likely got traveler's diarrhea. If you can, see a physician to confirm the diagnosis. In Mexico you often can go directly to the pharmacist and get antibacterial medication over the counter. Often a 3-day course of fluoroquinolones (e.g. Cipro), trimethoprim-sulfamethoxazole, azithromycin, or rifaximin is effective.

Whether the antibiotic is effective depends on the area where you travel, which also determines the resistance pattern. Further, it depends on what organisms are present in the contaminated food or environment, and it depends on the patient's age. For children below 16 the recommended antibiotic is azithromycin, for persons older than 16 ciprofloxacin (Cipro) is used.

Prevention of food poisoning

We can do a lot to avoid food poisoning. First of all, we need to wash our hands after having used the washroom and before we handle food. Avoid cross contamination as already described. Wash your hands again when you are finished handling raw meat, particularly hamburger meat. Make sure that meat is cooked until it is completely done. You may want to use a food thermometer, which will assist you to know that the meat is thoroughly cooked. Pork is done at 140°F, but chicken and ground poultry should be cooked until the meat temperature reaches 165°F. Ground beef requires 160°F. It is safer to include a 3-minute rest time following the reaching of the target temperature to ensure that no more live bacteria or viruses are left in the cooked meat.

Conclusion

Have a safe summer and enjoy backyard BBQ's following the simple rules mentioned before. Should you travel, make sure to be vigilant about food safety. Drink bottled water and brush your teeth with bottled water. Stick to a simple rule: if you can peel it, you can eat it. These measures will help you prevent traveler's diarrhea. The principles of safe food handling and food preparation are simple and can be learnt by anyone. Make sure that any unused food is refrigerated right after the meal, not more than two hours later. Food that has been sitting around on the buffet table or the kitchen counter for several hours may not be smelly; it may look perfectly fine, but the bacteria will have done their invisible work. Get rid of it; it's better to be safe than sorry!

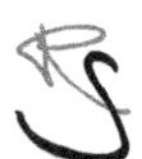

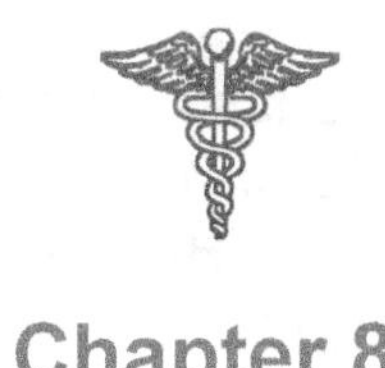

Chapter 8:

Healthy Limbs and Joints

We likely underestimate the importance of the strength of our limbs and joints. We need a good physical frame with muscles, tendons and working joints in order to balance properly and move about. Children and adolescents hardly ever have a problem with this unless there are sports injuries or other accidents. But in later middle age and old age major problems can set in. In the following paragraphs I will review the impact of arthritis and what can be done about it. One section will deal with the fact that a study has found a lower mortality in old age with a higher muscle mass. Unfortunately the opposite is usually true: high mortality due to lower muscle mass. Finally, the use of prolotherapy and stem cell therapy will be discussed, very useful newer methods to cure musculoskeletal problems.

Arthritis

Arthritis is an illness of the joints, mostly in older people (osteoarthritis or degenerative arthritis). However, a subgroup of younger patients can also develop a severe form of arthritis, called rheumatoid arthritis where autoimmune antibodies play more of a role.

In the 1950's Dan Dale Alexander wrote a book called "Arthritis and common sense". The medical establishment did not accept that simple remedy and Dan Dale Alexander was classified as a "quack". However, Dr. Mirkin describes a study from Berlin that later confirmed that Dan Dale Alexander's observation was correct: an emulsion made by shaking orange juice with cod liver oil and taken three times per day on an empty stomach would indeed improve osteoarthritis.

In 1964, still being a medical student I suggested to my future mother-in-law to give Dan Dale Alexander's book about arthritis a try. Despite the well-established osteoarthritic condition in her left knee the arthritis vanished within 6 months and stayed controlled. I could not explain to her why this remedy worked, as higher doses of omega-3 fatty acids and higher doses of vitamin C were not yet known to be of value for arthritis.

This all changed with the advent of orthomolecular medicine. Dr. Frederick Klenner describes that ascorbic acid (vitamin C) at mega doses of at least 10,000 mg daily, but better even between 15,000 and 25,000 mg daily does have healing effects on arthritis. He stated further that repair of collagenous tissue (the joint surfaces) would require adequate ascorbic acid. Dr. Abram Hoffer, the founder of modern orthomolecular medicine reviewed the history of the use of vitamins in higher doses, particularly the use of vitamin B3 (niacin). He also mentioned that Dr. William Kaufman had used mega doses of vitamin B3 for arthritis as far back as 1950.

Overview of arthritis

Dr. Hoffer explains that arthritis belongs into a group of diseases that are related to faulty nutrition, which in turn lead to vitamin and mineral deficiencies and a pandeficiency disease. Other diseases that belong to that group are cardiovascular disease, multiple sclerosis, cancer, diabetes, schizophrenia, mood disorders, alcoholism and autism. Contributing factors can be poor diets with overemphasis on refined and processed foods and consumption of sugar, allergies, diseases of the gastrointestinal tract and viral infections. Arthritis belongs into this group of illnesses as well. Niacin, vitamin B6 and zinc have been found useful to treat arthritis, but other vitamins and minerals are also needed. Here is a list of what Dr. Hoffer suggested to use:

1. Vitamin B3 from 100 mg to several thousand mg three times daily following meals. With niacin there can be skin flushing, which often goes away after the body gets used to the higher doses; but niacinamide could be used instead by those who are bothered by the flushing.

2. B complex: This contains each of the major B vitamins including vitamin B6 (pyridoxine). Take 100 mg once per day with a meal. Vitamin B6 may be needed up to 500 mg per day or more.

3. Vitamin C should be taken between 500 mg and several thousand mg three times per day after meals.

4. Vitamin D3: 4000 IU per day in the summer months. In the winter months particularly populations who live far north require 6000 IU per day.

5. Vitamin B1 (thiamine): Alcoholics and very high sugar consumers need thiamine at 100 to 500 mg three times per day.

6. Folic acid at mega doses (prescription needed) works as an antidepressant, which requires 25 to 50 mg. To lower homocysteine levels lower doses of folic acid are sufficient.

7. Vitamin E: Usually 400 IU to 800 IU daily. Muscle wasting diseases, Huntington's disease and amyotrophic lateral sclerosis (ALS) require much higher doses up to 4000 IU per day.

8. Essential fatty acids (omega-3): It is strongly recommended to use a molecularly distilled product, which is free of mercury and PBC's at 1000 mg three times daily following meals.

9. Selenium: The required dosage is 200 to 600 micrograms once daily (with any meal). In areas where selenium is deficient, this is particularly important.

10. Zinc: 50 mg of zinc citrate or 220 mg of zinc sulfate once per day with a meal.

11. Calcium and magnesium: Dr. Hoffer suggested 1000 mg of calcium with 500 mg of magnesium, although many experts now say that 1000 mg of calcium with 1000 mg of magnesium may be better.

Dr. Hoffer pointed out that this program is compatible with any medication and is non-toxic.

Thoughts on treating arthritis

1. Conventional methods

The conventional approach to treatment of arthritis consists of nonsteroidal anti-inflammatory drugs (NSAIDs). Unfortunately NSAIDs have side effects like causing kidney damage after several years of use. Also, NSAIDs can lead to gastric bleeding from gastric erosions, which may require blood transfusions. Physiotherapy with reactivation and

swimming has been found to be useful. Electro acupuncture can help for pain control. (Conventional treatment of arthritis).

2. Diet changes, multivitamins and minerals

As arthritis is found mostly in civilized nations, dietary factors have long been suspected to be of importance. Dr. Hoffer pointed out that arthritis is a pandeficiency disease meaning that overconsumption of sugar and processed foods has lead to multiple vitamin and mineral deficits that interfere with the cartilage metabolism leading to premature break-down of cartilage and causing inflammation. It is not good enough to just take the supplements listed above; this needs to be combined with a fundamental change in diet. Cut out sugar and starchy foods. Return to homemade foods. Keep it simple with lots of vegetables, salads and organic meats. Now that you are starting to turn around your metabolism by a sensible diet the supplements listed above have a chance to work.

You will notice that Dan Dale Alexander's idea of omega-3 fatty acids and vitamin C from the freshly pressed orange juice is contained in the list of supplements above. Dr. Klenner's mega doses of vitamin C are also listed and Dr. Kaufman's mega doses of vitamin B3 is contained in Dr. Hoffer's list as well.

This list may not have been formally researched with controlled clinical trials, because the food industry and the makers of NSAIDs (Big Pharma) have no interest in this. But thousands of patients have been empirically treated with this regimen and a network of orthomolecular physicians has established that this regimen works to control the inflammation of arthritis and there are no toxic side effects from it.

3.Laser, platelet rich plasma (PRP) and stem cells

Blue and green low-dose lasers have anti-inflammatory properties and are suitable for interstitial and intraarticular laser treatments for arthritis. Dr. Weber has extensive experience with this treatment modality in Germany. I am discussing the use of low-dose laser phototherapy by Dr. Weber in cancer patients under chapter 10 below.

However, prolotherapy, PRP and stem cell treatments are also an option for more severe cases of arthritis, particularly in arthritis of the knees, which can avoid total knee replacement surgery (see "Prolotherapy and stem cell therapy" below).

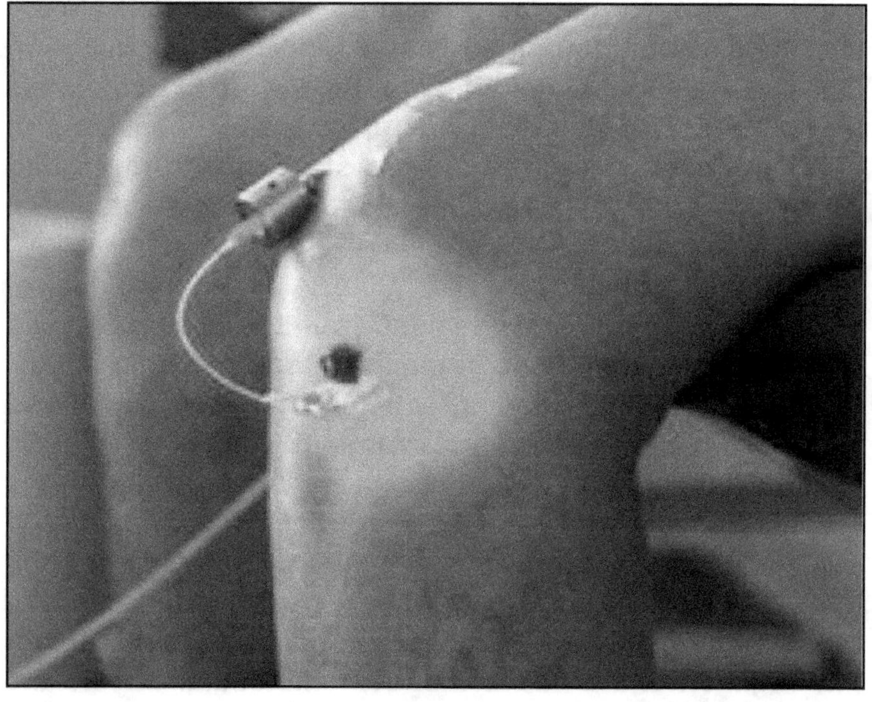

Image courtesy of Dr. Michael Weber, author of : "Medical Low-Level-Lasertherapy - Foundations and Clinical Applications", Amazon 2016 (ISBN 978-3-00-050017-6)

Conclusion

I met Dr. Hoffer in the early 1980's during a meeting in Vancouver, BC when he wanted to establish a local orthomolecular division for British Columbia, Canada. Although I found the ideas fascinating, I felt that the College of Physicians and Surgeons (the regulatory body for physicians in BC) would scrutinize the practice of any orthomolecular member. At that time I would risk losing my license to practice medicine, which I just had received in 1978. So I decided not to join. Interestingly enough later in the 1980's a member of the orthomolecular society of BC lost his license because of the use of mega doses of intravenous vitamin C. At this time the College considered these infusions useless or hazardous. Nowadays, any naturopathic and orthomolecular physician uses these intravenous vitamin C treatments as standard therapies. It shows how times have changed.

What has not changed is the food industry that undermines our health every day with hidden sugar contained in processed foods. In social functions it is customary to have a drink or two, if not more, which uses up our thiamine faster than we can replace it. Pandeficiency disease is alive and well as it was many years ago. It is in front of our eyes, but can we see it? Depending on what your eating habits are you may need to make changes in your diet and perhaps take some or all of the ingredients of the multivitamin and mineral list above? Start by adopting a Mediterranean type diet; next add some of the supplements listed above. It is time to take a thorough look at prevention and natural treatment modalities against arthritis in the interest of preserving your health!

Keep your muscles in older age

Intuitively you may have noted that older folks who have very little "meat" on them are not as healthy as people of the same age with well-developed muscles.

A research team under the supervision of Dr. Preethi Srikanthan and Dr. Arun S. Karlamangla from the David Geffen School of Medicine at UCLA, Los Angeles, CA decided to measure the muscle mass index instead of the body mass index. They did this using bioelectrical impedance (simple electronic body composition bathroom scales) and they wanted to see whether there would be any correlation with regard to mortality statistics in an older population.

The study group consisted of 3659 participants from the National Health and Nutrition Examination Survey III (average age for males 55 and older, females 65 and older). The survey took place between 1988-1994. The mortality rates were computed by the end of 2004. The median length of follow-up per person was 13.2 years.

The authors of the study compared mortality curves for four subgroups of muscle mass from low to high: 0-25%, 26-50%, 51 to 75% and 76 to 100%. When the lowest muscle mass group was compared to the highest muscle mass group, there was a 20% increased mortality rate for the lowest muscle mass group.

This study had careful controls built in and could demonstrate that the difference was not due to better or worse LDL cholesterol values or triglycerides; it was not due to differences in diabetic rates or other factors. This is the first study that shows in a US based population that a lower than average muscle mass is an independent risk factor for premature death in an older population.

The authors were aware of a Danish study that had previously shown that a lower muscle mass was associated with a higher mortality rate in 50 to 64 year-olds.

I like to comment regarding this study by putting it into the context of other medical findings.

1. Older people tend to have more falls

Several studies have shown over the years that older people fall more often because of a combination of balance problems with slower reaction time, and also because of poorer muscle development when compared to a younger age group. The medical costs are staggering when older people reach the age of 85, where about 20% of that subpopulation experience serious falls resulting in hip fractures and hospitalizations. There is a mortality of about 25% associated with hip fractures in that age group. About 50% of those who survive will not be living independently one year following a hip fracture. Fortunately fractures from falls can largely be prevented by making physical changes to the home to prevent tripping and having extra guard rails where needed. But another important factor is to exercise regularly within the capabilities of the older person to maintain muscle mass, which will balance the body and control upper and lower extremity strength. This is important for the person to move around safely.

2. Fit people live longer

A Stanford University study followed 6000 middle-aged men for 10 years and found that the fittest who exercised regularly were 12% more likely to stay alive for every metabolic equivalent; this is the energy that a sitting person uses in terms of oxygen consumption. They also found that the least fit had a 4.5-fold higher death rate within 6 years from the beginning of the study when compared to the fittest group.

To put this into perspective: a regular walk at less than two miles an hour would be equivalent to 2 metabolic equivalents, a brisk walk at 4 miles per hour is worth 5 metabolic equivalents and running 6 miles an hour is worth 8 metabolic equivalents. This is how the math works: a regular walk every day translates into 2×12% = 24% more likelihood of staying alive in the next 6 years compared to a sedentary person. A person exercising with a brisk walk with a speed of 4 miles per hour every day would be 5×12% = 60% more likely to be alive in 6 years compared to a sedentary person who does not exercise. Not smoking and having a normal weight would also add to your probability of living longer. Pushing yourself to the extreme like running 6 miles per hour or going on marathon runs may be problematic for the majority of us as adrenal gland insufficient can develop, if you over-stress yourself. This is my comment, not part of the study.

Now you may have wondered about the woman's side, as the previous study was an all-male study. The answer comes from a recent paper that studied 10 clinical trials throughout the world (US, Denmark, Germany, Sweden, Taiwan, Japan and others) involving only postmenopausal women. Yes, there is the same surprising finding that regular brisk exercise makes the women live longer with less disabilities and less mortality!

The bottom line for both men and women is: exercise regularly and live.

3. Exercise develops your muscles and maintains them

We were born to use our muscles daily. We were basically designed as hunter and gatherers, but in the meantime this is what we do: sitting in front of the computer or TV, in cars, in class (school, university, work) or in the movie theater. So we need to discipline ourselves to get into a routine that balances all of the other activities. Muscle strength exercises or activities are the answer.

The earlier we adopt this type of a routine, the better off we are when we reach the golden years of retirement. I am one of the examples of former non-exercisers. Apart from liking to go for long walks 3 to 4 times per week I did no formal exercises until 2005 when my wife and I got into ballroom and Latin dancing inspired by "Dancing with the stars". But it is only since 2012 that we took up regular gym workouts for 45 to 60 minutes every day on top of a regular dance program. It is now easier for me to walk up on a steep hill in our neighborhood that has an 18% incline than before 2012. Muscles need regular exercise. You put a limb in a cast and within 3 weeks most of the muscle strength has melted away. You remove the cast, and it will take 3 to 6 weeks of regular exercise to regain the muscle strength. So why not maintain your muscle strength in the first place?

4. Exercise develops cardiovascular fitness

The aerobic part of my daily exercise program (treadmill) develops cardiovascular fitness as the lungs have to work harder and the heart is being activated. But this is not engraved in stone: some people relate to an elliptical machine or a stair master. Doing this regularly is mimicking going through the landscape looking for food and hunting. Of course most of us drive in our cars to the grocery store and get our food that way. So my balance is to go to the gym and at least once a day get that workout. What can we expect from fitness training? An NIH study showed that with a moderate workout of only 2.5 hours per week you would gain 4.5 years of life due to cardiovascular fitness. This is better than money in the account. It is free healthy additional life!

5. Sensible nutrition will help preserve muscle mass

No, I am not taking your food away. I am suggesting that we watch the quality of the food we are consuming. If you are like the average consumer, you may be eating too many carbs in form of pasta, bread, rice and potatoes. Some of you have read in past blogs on my website www.askdrray.com that my wife and I cut out sugar and starchy foods as well as wheat since 2001. We both lost 50 pounds and kept it down. I know that if I would restart sugar and starchy foods, my fat content would go up, my muscle content down and the BMI up. How do I know? I weigh myself every day on body composition scales (which works by the principal of bioelectrical impedance analysis). This shows all of these indicators. In the summer of 2014 I got into some organic Bing cherries. They were delicious, but they are also a fruit with significant sugar content! Within a day I knew that I'd better watch the quantities of cherries I consume as my fat composition was up and, my muscles mass was down. It took 3 days for my values to be back to normal.

When it comes to muscle mass, overconsumption of refined carbs is one problem; however, our bodies do need quality lean meat and some fish (salmon, mackerel; low mercury fish) as a source of protein. I buy organic meats to get away from the problem of pesticide pollution and antibiotic residues as much as possible. Some people like vegetarian or vegan food, they may need to supplement with protein supplements.

6. Human growth hormone deficiency

In some people when they age the reason for a lack of muscle mass may be an age-related lack of growth hormone (GH) production of the pituitary gland. Dr. Hertoghe, an endocrinologist from Belgium gave a lecture at the 23rd Annual World Congress on Anti-Aging Medicine on Dec.

13, 2015 in Las Vegas that I attended. He talked about the life-prolonging effect of human growth hormone. He explained that he has done blood tests (IGF-1) and lately also 24-hour urine metabolite tests of growth hormone on aging patients and found that many are deficient with regard to GH production. These were patients who already had their thyroid hormones replaced, if abnormal and had their sex hormones replaced when they were found to be low. But they lost hair, developed old looking faces with wrinkles, loss of subcutaneous fatty tissue giving the face a hollow appearance. They also had muscle and joint pains and thin skin, particularly over the back of their hands. He replaced their missing GH using daily GH self-injections with a tiny needle (similar to diabetes injections) and within 1.5 to 3 years the wrinkles disappeared, the faces started to look younger and patients did feel younger. Their muscle and joint pains had disappeared and their hair grew back. The dosage range is between 0.1mg and 0.3mg, a tiny amount of GH daily. This is not inexpensive, but some health care plans pay for this, as a lack of GH is a true hormone deficiency. Dr. Hertoghe said that according to his research the normalization of growth hormone levels would add between 19 and 34 years (average 26.5 years) of healthy life to these previously frail patients. A large effect of this is the restoration of joint mobility and the building up of muscle mass from replacing missing human growth hormone.

Conclusion

It may sound like common sense that a body with well-developed muscles will live longer. You may want to compare this to a well-maintained car. With proper maintenance the car will still drive well once it has a high mileage.

We have bodies that need maintenance (exercise) and good nutrition (no junk food, but a sensible diet like the

Mediterranean diet). If we make this our regular lifestyle, we will develop and maintain muscles. It will keep us in the group with a lower mortality rate compared to sessile persons and junk food consumers.

Nothing happens without any effort. We need to earn muscle fitness for ourselves! Think about it, improve where you need to improve, and then maintain it. More than anything else this will pay dividends well into your future.

Prolotherapy and stem cell therapy

Chronic back pain, joint pains and arthritis are among the conditions that respond to prolotherapy and stem cell therapy. If you have any of these chronic pain conditions you know how difficult it is to exercise to keep fit.

Prolotherapy and stem cell therapy were among the topics discussed at the 22nd Annual Anti-Aging Conference in Las Vegas (Dec.10 to 14, 2014). Here are summaries of two talks from this conference that dealt with methods of repairing damage to your joints or bones without surgery. Treatments consist of stimulating local stem cells through a treatment called "prolotherapy" where needles are used to inject concentrated dextrose. I will explain below why this method is effective. A modification of this original prolotherapy consists of amplifying it through growth factors from so-called platelet rich plasma (PRP), which is mixed with the dextrose injection. The ultimate healing jerk occurs when you mix in stem cells with the PRP into the injured tissues. Images before the procedures and images some time after the procedures were shown at both lectures with impressive results.

1. Dr. Fields' talk was entitled "Repairing joints and spine without surgery: prolotherapy/PRP/stem cell therapy".

This talk concentrated on the use of prolotherapy with concentrated dextrose and prolotherapy with platelet rich plasma (PRP) with or without the addition of stem cells in the treatment of various musculoskeletal injuries.

When prolotherapy is done by itself 12.5% Dextrose is used to inject into the area of injury. Dr. Fields said that the reason it works is that local stem cells in the injured area are getting activated where Dextrose is injected, and these activated stem cells will do the healing. This result can be improved by injecting a small amount of PRP very focally to an area of ligament rupture. PRP is obtained by centrifuging blood from the patient's vein, which allows separating the platelet rich plasma. The red blood cells are discarded, but the platelet fraction and some of the plasma is used as the PRP preparation. To amplify the effect of the PRP, stem cells from bone marrow and from fatty tissue are mixed into the injection. Dr. Fields explained that bone marrow is aspirated from the pelvic bone and in the same patient a liposuction is also done to receive adipose tissue. Both tissue samples are put through a cell separator to obtain bone marrow derived stem cells and adipose derived mesenchymal stem cells. Both fractions are combined, as they make a superior stem cell mix and are activated by adding platelet rich plasma. This mix was used for bone fractures that were slow to heal, for ruptured tendons, ligaments, Achilles tendons and rotator cuff tears. Dr. Fields showed before-slides and several weeks to months after-slides with MRI scans of the original injuries and the final healed tendons and ligaments. I have never seen such beautiful healing with no residual scar. Stem cells are the specialists of healing such defects because they change into whatever cell type is required and they fill in the defects without scar formation. Function of the area will be restored after the injury is healed following stem cell and PRP injection. It also explains why many athletes who had this done could win more medals after such a repair. You do not hear much about success stories following conventional surgery, because range of motion and strength suffer from the scarring after conventional surgical repairs.

Case histories

Several patients with knee injuries that were treated with prolotherapy were shown on video testimonials explaining that their procedures only involved needles in the injured area, that they experienced almost complete pain relief on the day of the procedure, and that they could rehabilitate right away.

Slides were also shown of specific knee ligament injuries involving the medial collateral ligament (MCL), the posterior cruciate ligament (PCL) and the anterior cruciate ligament (ACL). These are very important support ligaments within the knee.

But this was not all: there were lower back injuries with ruptured discs. Conventional medicine would have offered a discectomy, but here these patients were treated with prolotherapy. They experienced a stabilization of the weak areas, spontaneous resorption of the prolapsed disc and stabilization and strengthening of the weak spine. MRI scans of the spinal injury before treatment and several months after the treatment were shown with a complete normalization of the spine. In my work as a Medical Advisor for Workers' Compensation over a 16 year period I have never seen a single case like that.

A similar spinal injury in the neck was shown as well with a testimonial from that person. Again there was minimal pain, immediate rehabilitation and a full range of motion several weeks after the injury had been treated with stem cells and PRP prolotherapy.

What is treated with prolotherapy?

Basically all of the major joints can be treated with prolotherapy: the shoulder, knee, back, the neck, ankle, elbow and hip. The types of injuries that are treated are sports injuries, fibromyalgia, sciatica, muscle tears, tendonitis, arthritis, bursitis and temporomandibular joint problems (TMJ).

Dr. Fields also stressed (and so did Dr. Purita) that activated platelet rich plasma (activated PRP) needs to be used to activate stem cells.

Two special cases were presented, namely patellar tendinitis and Achilles tendinitis, which both responded very well to prolotherapy and PRP plus stem cell therapy. This provides complete healing of these otherwise very difficult clinical entities.

An image was shown from the late C. Everett Koop, MD, the former Surgeon General of the United States who had this to say about prolotherapy: "I have been a patient who has benefited from prolotherapy. Having been so remarkably relieved of my chronic disabling pain, I began to use it on some of my patients." This may yet be the strongest argument to at least consider prolotherapy in otherwise hopeless cases.

2. Dr. Joseph Purita gave a lecture on the "Effects of PRP And Stem Cell Injections". Dr. Purita is an orthopedic surgeon who now specializes in regenerative medicine. As explained above PRP stands for platelet rich plasma, which is a "soup" of various growth factors. He discussed the importance of the proper harvesting of PRP. He explained that apart from white blood cells (WBC) and platelets an important component of PRP are very small embryonic like stem cells (VSELs). They can be seen under the microscope. The missing link has been the observation that white blood

cells produce inflammatory substances, which have been detrimental when stem cell injections with PRP were done in the past, which led to poor survival rates of stem cells.

Now it has been detected that photo-activation of the PRP before injection leads to anti-inflammatory behavior of the WBC in PRP. Dr. Purita calls this "light activated PRP", which leads to the best results with stem cell/PRP injections. Soft laser stimulation with red, green and blue soft lasers have been shown to improve tissue healing significantly when stem cells and light activated PRP are used with the Dr. Weber laser system. Dr. Purita showed very detailed technical aspects of these procedures with various applications. For instance, he showed a slide regarding treatment for osteoarthritis of the knee. Light activated PRP is injected into a joint with degenerative arthritis. When you mix this with bone and adipose tissue derived stem cells and inject it into the knees of a person with degenerative arthritis, you get the ideal remedy to calm down the degenerative process with instant pain relief, and the stem cells are transforming into cartilage cells (chondrocytes) building up hyaline cartilage. The end result is a new knee surface where the old and the new repaired knee surfaces are knitted into one seamless unit. Conventional surgery cannot achieve this!

Towards the end of the talk Dr. Purita showed an MRI scan of a knee with avascular necrosis (dead bone) before and after treatment with stem cells, PRP and low-level laser therapy. There was a complete resolution of the avascular necrosis without any surgery. A second case was shown where the initial MRI scan showed a complete tear of the medium collateral ligament (MCL tear) of the knee, and the follow-up scan showed the same ligament intact. This was achieved with a non-invasive procedure, without surgery, just by treating the patient with an injection of stem cells, and low-level laser therapy activated PRP.

Conclusion

Prolotherapy and stem cell therapy are the hottest new treatment modalities for ruptured tendons, ligamentous injuries, and disc herniations in the neck and in the lower back. You will not get this from your primary care physician or from your regular orthopedic surgeon at the present time; unfortunately the profit motive associated with the conventional procedures is a barrier towards progress. But you owe it to your health to try these alternatives first as they are much less invasive and they involve your own cells that will heal the defects with a very high probability. You still have the option to seek the advice of an orthopedic surgeon, should these alternative procedures fail (which is unlikely). Unfortunately most insurance carriers will not pay for prolotherapy, PRP or stem cell therapy at this time.

Using the links given in the references section, you can view before and after pictures.

Disclaimer: Dr. Schilling has no conflict of interest with regard to Regenexx or any of the other companies of which images are shown under references; they simply displayed the best images with regard to the many illustrations in this section.

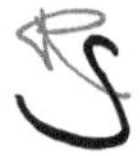

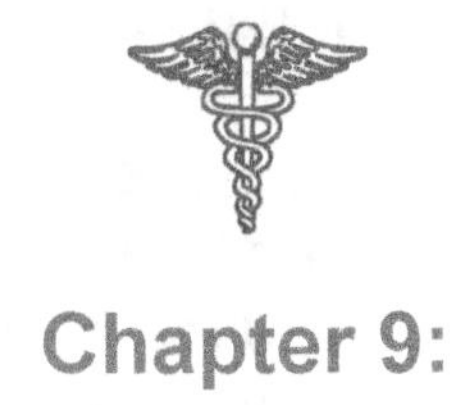

Chapter 9:

Keep Toxins Out

Toxins lurk around us more than we know: they are in the air as pollution, which we inhale; they are also in the water, but we cannot necessarily taste it. Noxious substances are worked into processed foods, milk, wheat, but in different forms. I cannot cover every aspect of toxins here; this would be an entire book. What I will cover are environmental toxins, molds, lead poisoning, and radioactivity. I will also discuss the use of chelation therapy for detoxification.

Environmental toxins

Environmental toxins are toxins that may be in your drinking water, in what you eat, they may be in the air you breathe, or they enter your body through your skin when you swim in contaminated water or walk on a sandy, wet beach.

The following discussion will address some of these issues and how we can defend ourselves against toxins.

The youngest and most vulnerable

Toxins are particularly bad for infants and premature babies. Here are the reasons: their kidney function (tubular secretion) is only 20% to 30% of that of an adult; the cytochrome P-450 enzyme system in the liver, one of the toxin eliminators is slowed down to only 25% to 50% of the adult activity, and glucuronidation in the liver, another detoxification process, reaches adult levels only at the age of 3 years. The kidneys and the liver are limiting the removal of toxins by way of urine and bile in the newborn. Stomach acidity in a premature has a pH of 4.7, in a full-term newborn 2.3–3.6 and in an adult 1.4–2.0. This is important to note as a lack of stomach acid increases susceptibility of newborns and infants to gastrointestinal infections and can cause diarrhea. Due to the tender skin of babies, absorption through the skin in newborns is much higher than in adults, which makes them very susceptible to skin absorption of toxins.

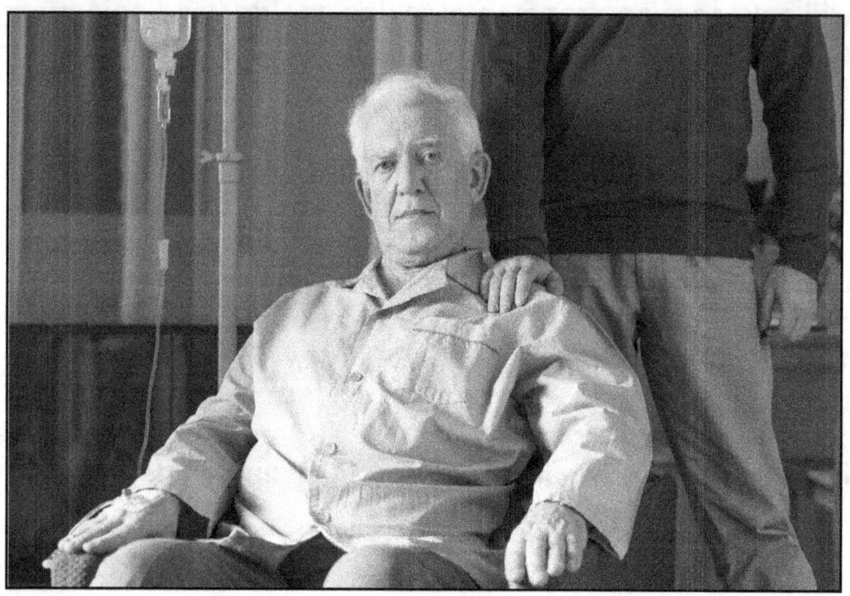

Diabetes from environmental toxins

Environmental toxins can cause insulin resistance and type 2 diabetes.

Bisphenol A (BPA) is used to make polycarbonate and epoxy resins and is found primarily in food and beverage containers. The world population has been exposed to this since 1957 and as a result 90% of US residents have detectable levels of BPA in their urine. The higher the urine concentration of BPA, the higher the risk is for developing diabetes.

Persistent organic pollutants are another source of concern: pesticides and herbicides, dioxins, polychlorinated biphenyls, hexachlorobenzene, and hexachlorocyclohexane have all been found in humans. Several investigators have shown that virtually all of the risk in obese patients to develop diabetes comes from the fat-soluble persistent organic pollutants.

Inorganic arsenic is another pollutant that is found in soil and rock naturally and finds its way into the drinking water. About 8% of the public water system of the US exceeds arsenic levels of 10 mcg/L for drinking water, which has been set as the safe limit by the US Environmental Protection Agency's standard. Anything above those levels is considered toxic. Rakel describes that people who ingest inorganic arsenic will excrete it in the urine; the highest group with arsenic in their urine had a risk of 3.58-fold to develop diabetes when compared to the lowest group. Curiously enough organic arsenic that is found in fish and shellfish is excreted in the urine unchanged and does not cause diabetes. Overall this indicates to me that nobody should consume or cook with contaminated water that contains inorganic arsenic. Reverse osmosis filters will protect you from this risk. Otherwise purified drinking water should be purchased.

Other toxins around the house

Volatile organic compounds are often contained in carpets, but also in laser and inkjet printers. They are part of everyone's life. Varied symptoms like irritation of eyes, nose or throat, breathing problems, headaches, loss of coordination, damage to the liver, kidneys and the brain have been reported after exposure to volatile organic compounds. Long-term exposure can even cause cancer in animals and has been suspected to cause cancer in humans as well.

Air fresheners and cleaning solutions that contain ethylene-based glycol ethers and terpenes have been the subject of a study that examined concentrations in the air and interaction with ozone that can also be released by some cleaners. The investigators concluded that with exposure to high enough concentrations and long-time exposures to these fumes lung cancer can be caused in cleaning personnel. They recommended using cleaning solutions only in diluted form and to air out the premises well after cleaning. Another component of many air fresheners and cleaning chemicals is paradichlorobenzene, the same chemical that is contained in mothballs and one of the "10 dangerous everyday things".

There have been problems with flame retardants: polybrominated diphenyl ethers, which are cancer producing; they have been outlawed in the US since 2004, but older mattresses, upholstery, television, computer casings and circuit boards may still contain them.

Lead and mercury poisoning, and radioactive pollutants

Manufacturers were not allowed to use lead in paints anymore since 1978. Paint from buildings older than that still may contain lead. There have been serious lead poisonings in children who were gnawing on items painted with lead containing paint. Lead causes problems with your central nervous system, brain, blood cells and kidneys. In 2012 a news story about lead found in fashion jewelry surfaced, warning about cheap fashion jewelry from China. Lead from these items can be absorbed through the skin and cause lead poisoning. Because of the apparent lack of regulations in China it is my recommendation not to buy anything that goes into your mouth or on your skin, if it has been grown or produced in China.

Heavy metals like mercury are found in tuna and other predator fish: it is sad that the oceans are polluted to the point where it has become unsafe to eat predator fish, as there is an accumulation of mercury through the food chain.

How did things develop this way? Back 100 years ago gold panning and the purification process of gold caused mercury to enter into rivers and allow mercury to end up in the oceans where it has since accumulated; it just sits there as it has nowhere to go.

There is also mercury in coal. Coal burning has contributed to mercury pollution of air by smoke being emitted from smoke stacks containing mercury vapors. The mercury vapors ended up returning to earth as polluted rain and drained through the river system into the oceans.

It is monomethylmercury that accumulates in the tissue of humans. It affects many organs, such as the brain, kidneys, lungs, and skin. It causes various symptoms like red cheeks, fingers, and toes; there can be bleeding from the mouth and ears; it can cause rapid heartbeats, high blood pressure, intense sweating, loss of hair, teeth, and nails. It also can cause blindness, loss of hearing, impaired memory, and lack of coordination, disturbed speech and birth defects. You may think all mercury comes from the outside. However, silver amalgam fillings in your teeth could also be a source of mercury poisoning from the inside. It is a good idea to replace amalgam/mercury fillings with ceramic fillings.

There are many forms of other marine pollution as well as you can find in the reference section.

One particular concerning aspect is pollution with radioactive materials as the Fukushima disaster in Japan has shown. Following the catastrophe on March 11, 2011 there have been several leaks of radioactive material into the ocean. The book by Dr. John Apsley II points out that with the explosions in Fukushima several releases of radioactive pollution into the stratosphere occurred. This pollution has subsequently traveled around the globe and has come down as radioactive rain. He has made it his ambition to help people minimize radiation exposure from nuclear accidents such as Fukushima.

Protecting yourself from toxins

Having said that pollution and toxins are problems that we are living with, how can we protect ourselves from all of that?

1. Avoid as many unsafe chemicals around you as you can. This includes checking ingredients in hair care and body care products, toothpaste, hair dyes, cosmetics, mouthwashes and underarm deodorants. I have written a blog about toxins in the bathroom and what you should watch out for (link under references).

2. I would recommend you switch from standard food to organic food. It has become unsafe to eat non-organic meats, leafy vegetables, vegetables and fruit. Also there are

too many residues of herbicides and pesticides contained in meat, vegetables and fruit. Washing will not remove these substances, even though some merchants may tell you otherwise. Buyer beware!

3. Detoxification methods are available and I have reviewed them in a blog with the heading "Get rid of toxins safely" (see references). Briefly, to remove lead and mercury a formal intravenous chelation protocol should be followed. Depending on how many heavy metal toxins you have on board, you may need only a few treatments or else up to 20. The popular website WebMD is still stating that it would be safe to have silver amalgam fillings. I disagree and think that gold and ceramic fillings are much safer.

4. Genetically modified food is another danger as I have summarized in a blog entitled "Living in a toxic world" (see references). This is another reason why I like to stick to organic foods. There is evidence that GMO food causes autoimmune diseases, infertility and chronic inflammation that can eventually lead to cancer. It may take decades to prove this, but I am not willing to be a human guinea pig.

5. You also need to carefully look at your home and remove toxins. You need to assess your drinking water. A water analysis can tell you more about the water quality in your home and whether there are concerns about inorganic arsenic. Usually places that sell filter systems can advise you in that regard. Your drinking water should either be bottled pure water or else reverse osmosis water that can be part of a filter system in your house.

6.Vitamins and supplements have been shown to support your cell integrity and have anti-inflammatory and antioxidant effects that protect you from toxins. I discussed this in detail in my website NetHealthBook.com under "Vitamins, minerals and supplements". For instance vitamin D3 in doses of 5000 IU or more and CoQ-10 are powerful anti-inflammatories and CoQ-10 is an antioxidant that preserves mitochondrial cell function. High fish oil supplements (3 to 6 Grams per day) have anti-inflammatory effects and protect your cell membrane integrity. With these overlapping qualities of vitamins and supplements your body will be in a much stronger position to defend itself against the negative effects of toxins. When you take multivitamins, this translates into telomere lengthening of 5.1% or converted into a survival advantage of 9.8 years when it is accumulated over a lifetime. Xu et al. have researched this in 2009.

7. Exposure to radioactive substances is a scary thought, but this is becoming more and more a reality, at least for those who live close to disaster areas such as the Fukushima site in Japan or the Chernobyl site in the Ukraine. But according to Dr. Apsley II low dose radiation that we have already received in the US and in Canada following the Fukushima disaster is equally disastrous. Many of the vitamins and supplements I have mentioned are also cell and mitochondria protective and will help with DNA repair following radiation damage, but you must avoid sugar and other refined carbs and starches to reduce the oxidative effect on cells and on LDL cholesterol to prevent premature aging and cell death. A lot more detail can be found in Dr. Apsley's book about this and what specific supplements you can take to detoxify your system from radioactive substances. This text also explains that there are specific antidotes for radioactive iodine-129 and iodine-131, radioactive cesium-137 and others.

Conclusion

Many people shrug their shoulders when they hear that pollution has an effect on their lives. They feel that they are powerless and cannot do anything about this. The truth is far from this! I have mentioned seven points above that you can follow to counter toxins. On top of that you can get politically active and urge your government representative to create a nuclear free zone in your area. Dr. Apsley's book contains compelling evidence why this is so important not only for us now, but for future generations and the future of mankind. We need to hold those who provide us with food and beverages accountable for the quality of these. Shrugging it off is not good enough. Get involved. Buy organic food. Avoid the section in the grocery store where sugar and high carb foods are sold. It's good for your own health, but it will also collectively change the mentality of the grocery store owners who will notice that they are stuck with the so-called comfort foods that sold well in the past. This new trend will result in more affordable prices for healthy foods and more availability of organic food.

Mold allergies

In a recent news story ("Moldy dream home") extensive mold infestation was found in a house that had oriented strand boards (OSB) instead of plywood walls. The house also was tightly sealed trapping moisture, which contributed to the extensive mold problem.

Mold problems have been around for centuries, but allergists have pointed out in the past few decades how important it is to prevent this from happening.

In the following I will review a few typical scenarios that can lead to mold accumulation.

1. Mold from airtight house construction

The homeowner described in the news story above is not the only case in the world that has a mold problem. Energy efficient homes are popular because they save energy costs; homeowners often also respond to gas companies, electric utility companies and government incentives to convert to airtight home construction.

In the 1980's the construction industry introduced the cheaper OSB products to replace the more expensive plywood for wall construction. This is frequently the problem with newer house construction. However, older homes are not immune to mold development.

2. Roof leaks in older homes

Older homes that were built in the 1970's may have plywood walls and have a bit of airflow from poorer wall construction, which would prevent mold formation. But roofs are older and do not always get replaced right away when a leak is detected. It may even take some time in areas where there is less precipitation before it is picked up during a particularly heavy rainstorm. Water that enters from a leaky roof can form a puddle on top of the ceiling where mold softens the drywall material until a leak in the ceiling causes water to drip down onto the floor. The mold spores multiply particularly well in wall-to-wall carpeting, but OSB material is also a good growth opportunity for molds due to the mini air spaces between the glued wood pieces. Plywood with its several tight layers is much more resistant to water penetration and mold growth.

3. Mold growth after hurricanes

After hurricane Sandy images of "black mold" were frequently shown in the media. The problem is that after 48

hours anything that has been in contact with water produces mold. However, often with disasters like hurricanes there are evacuation orders and the residents of the area cannot return to their homes for several days. There may be even further delays because there is a waiting period for insurers to assess the amount of damage, before the residents can even start with a clean up.

As a result of the delay it is not unusual that expensive mold sanitation is needed. In other cases the residents end up moving away, and the house is leveled before a new house can be built.

4. Effects of molds

People with preexisting allergies and asthma are more susceptible to the effects of molds. It leads to itchy eyes, wheezing, coughing, and exacerbation of asthma.

The CDC reviews how mold grows after a disaster. This website also explains that you can recognize a mold problem because of a musty smell or foul stench in the air and because of the appearance such as discoloration of ceilings or walls and signs of water damage.

You can clean hard surfaces with bleach water. Bleach kills molds, but it may have to be cleaned several times within a few days to get rid of the last spores. Whatever cannot be sanitized this way must be removed or replaced.

5. Health concerns regarding molds

Shannon's medical textbook on managing poisonings reviewed the public concern about the toxic effects of molds. It notes that with the Internet and the popular press having exaggerated some of the connections of symptoms with mold allergies, the term "mold madness" has been coined. Despite the paranoia in the general public about

toxins from molds, there is only a small percentage of the population that is sensitive to molds where IgE antibodies and IgG antibodies against molds can be determined through blood tests. These individuals often are also allergic to other environmental allergens like grass pollen and dust mites. The asthmatic reactions in sensitive people are not as severe as what peanut traces would do to peanut sensitive patients, but skin testing and blood test screening for specific IgE and IgG antibodies often do confirm that mold sensitive people indeed can have specific mold allergies. In the vast majority of people these tests are negative, and correlations between mold infestations and allergic reactions could not be verified.

6. Fixing mold damage and dealing with allergies

It follows from this that you should remove any visible mold and remedy whatever the cause was for its appearance. Carefully disinfect the areas with diluted bleach water (the CDC recommends 1 cup of bleach per 1 gallon of water) several times. Make sure the areas are dry and not musty; otherwise you have to work on improving ventilation. If you are not one of these hypersensitive persons, there is nothing further to worry about. However, if you are hypersensitive, an allergist should examine you. Common indoor molds that cause the so-called "immediate type hyper reactivity" are due to the mold species Aspergillum and Penicillium. Most outdoor molds that can cause problems for sensitive people are due to Alternaria and Cladosporium species. The latter would be the ones found in carpets after a leaky roof has caused problems. If the allergist has found specific allergies to one or several of the mold species, allergy shots may be prescribed. A sensitive person who has environmentally induced asthma would need allergy shots on a weekly basis. Often it takes several years for

these desensitization shots to stop the affected person from reacting to molds. In some cases patients need to stay on these allergy shots life-long.

Conclusion

The key with regard to mold allergies is to prevent mold growth by being vigilant about detecting early problems with leaky roofs, walls and cleaning up water damage right away. When there is a musty telltale smell, investigate right away and remedy the problem. For most people this is the end of the story. However, a small percentage of very sensitive people need to consult with an allergist who should investigate whether or not they would benefit from allergy injections.

In some rare cases the affected person may have to relocate to another house that has no mold infestation.

Lead still poisoning us

We are living in an environment that puts emphasis on quality control, and companies around us take pride in their high quality products, supervised by the FDA. This is how it should be. But is it really? Unfortunately not!

I read a headline about cosmetic products, namely lipsticks on April 4, 2014 and could not believe it!

When it comes to skin care or cosmetic products, things start to get scary in the bathroom. Our skin is not a barrier, but it is an organ of our body. From skin cream and ointment applications in medicine it is known that pharmaceutical compounds can be applied to the skin, and the body will readily absorb active substances through the skin.

The skin areas to which cosmetics are applied often have softer skin, for example, on the lips or around the eyes. The vulnerable skin of the lips can readily absorb any chemical substance, and this is where health concerns get even more serious.

In 2010 the FDA determined that all of the "400 lipsticks tested had traces of lead in them, ranging from 0.9 to 3.06 ppm". Another study from California noted that there were other toxic metals in lip sticks and lip glosses containing chromium, cadmium, manganese, and aluminum in addition to lead. Even to the unconcerned this sounds like a precarious cocktail of noxious substances! On June 1, 2013 I wrote a blog about toxins in the bathroom. I mentioned the dirty dozen of chemicals that repeatedly are found in cosmetics. With this new information about traces of lead still being in cosmetics, more so than previously reported, women need to be more careful about the choice of lipsticks that they are using.

1.History of lipsticks

This overview explains that the long-lasting lipstick was only invented around the 1950's. "Sticks on you, not on him" was the slogan at that time. Traces of lead were often recorded, but not really thought to be that dangerous. The Wikipedia has an interesting write-up about the "lipstick in the US". The thinking of the FDA at that time was that children needed to be protected from lead in house paints, but nobody mentioned that lead was part of the red pigment and therefore was part of a lipstick. The FDA did know this, but the concentration was supposed to be so small and absorption was thought to be negligible. It was considered to be safe for an adult.

2. Evidence of considerable absorption of lead

We know from several studies that various components of cosmetics including lipsticks and lip-glosses get absorbed through the skin. Lead is no exception to this.

A 2011 study of children in Africa showed that those who were exposed to lead-containing cosmetics for tribal ceremonies had higher lead concentrations in their blood than children who did not use these cosmetics.

When doing a PubMed review on the subject I came across a very interesting study: In India there is a practice to apply kajal (also called kohl or surma cosmetic) around the eyes, which is an old traditional practice. Unfortunately this is a lead-containing cosmetic, which is absorbed into the blood and can cause lead poisoning. According to an ancient belief this application of cosmetics around the eyes is supposed to keep the eyes cool and clean and is believed to improve vision, strengthen the eyes and prevent eye diseases. None of these beliefs are compatible with Western medicine, although a lot of the Ayurveda medicines are valid.

In another 2010 study done in the mountainous Aseer region in the Southwest of Saudi Arabia with pristine air quality, 176 pregnant patients with a single baby were followed to see whether there was an effect with regard to lead poisoning in the offspring. Two groups of women were identified, those with lead levels of more than 200 mcg/L in the blood and another group with less than 200 mcg/L. The researchers noted that there was no difference with regard to prematurity, size of the baby or premature rupture of membranes (premature birth).

Obviously air pollution is not a concern in this area. The lead came from a different source. The conclusion of this study was that there was significant absorption of lead from 100% lead sulfide eye cosmetic "kohl" only on those who used it. To my surprise nobody mentioned anything about the lead levels in the children, which is an example of compartmentalization of science. Common sense would dictate that the children from mothers with over 200 mcg/L who were at higher risk of lead poisoning should have

received chelation treatments to remove any accumulated lead. In Western medicine this is the treatment to get rid of lead poisoning.

3. Different lip sticks and lip glosses analyzed in Europe and in the US

A European study showed that 31% of lipsticks and 4% of lip-glosses tested positive for lead. All of them had less than 0.88 mg/kg of lead (less than 1 mg/kg). Pink lipstick or lip-gloss (0.81 and 0.38mg/kg) tested lower than purple lipstick or lip-gloss (0.88 and 0.37mg/kg) and red (0.58 and 0.25mg/kg), but purple tested the highest! On average the tests show that the gloss has half the concentration of the lipstick.

Don't be fooled by the difference in recommended safe levels in Canada (10 mg/kg) and Germany (20 mg/kg). Germany has a very powerful chemical industry with lobbyists that likely tolerate this higher "safe" level. In Canada it is the Health Products and Food Branch of Health Canada that watches. No country got it right so far: A zero tolerance (meaning a blood level of 0 mg/kg in babies and adults alike) is the only solution for humans. A little bit of lead over a long time can lead to chronic lead poisoning.

One other interesting tidbit for those who need to apply something to their lips:

The more expensive lipsticks had much less lead in it than the cheaper varieties. If you want to be safer, don't buy the discount store brands.

Contrast this to an FDA initiated study between 2009 and 2012, published in 2012 that showed that the average lipstick concentration in 400 lipsticks tested was 1.11 mg/kg, but the highest concentration was 7.19 mg/kg and 13 of them tested 3.06 mg/kg. Here is another review that shows more details (ppm equals mg/kg, so you can compare

directly with the figures above. As stated before, in my opinion and that of toxicologists around the world who are the real experts in this a "0 mg/kg" level (no lead in the body) should be the acceptable norm!

Only organic lipsticks and lip-glosses are recommended, if you wish to use any of such products. You can look up a helpful blog about "lead and chemical free lip products" that tells you more positive news (see references).

4. What are the effects of chronic low lead exposure?

Adult lead toxicity is not as common as in the past. Painters in the decades leading up to the 1970's when laws became more stringent were the ones mostly affected. Keep in mind that more than 30 million tons of lead was released into the air in the US before the lead ban finally remedied this in the 1970's. This phasing out was completed in 1995. Since then the mean blood lead levels of Americans have declined by 35%. The EPA is monitoring lead levels in public water systems.

Lead is a nerve poison. It leads to fatigue, insomnia, irritability, lethargy, headaches, difficulty concentrating, memory loss, and tremor. It can also affect the nerves of the extremities, more so in the arms than the legs, which was significant in the past century among painters using lead paints. According to Shannon's textbook on Poisoning and Drug Overdoses the symptoms of "upper extremity paresis" was typical for lead poisoning in painters before 1970. Chronic lead poisoning targets the kidneys and the bone marrow. In the kidneys leakage of the filtration units, called glomeruli, leads to loss of microglobulins that can be measured in the urine among other tests. Above a level of 30 mcg/dL (this is the same as above 300 mcg/L) electrophysiological studies reveal that the ulnar nerve conduction is slowed down, which is the cause for the arm weakness in painters. The bone marrow toxicity can be seen in stippling of red blood cells and anemia develops subsequently. High blood pressure and fertility issues are also common (low sperm count in men, higher rate of spontaneous abortions and stillbirths in women). The gums around the teeth show lead lines as a blue discoloration. I will not get into lead toxicity in children, as this is a big topic of its own. Needless to say, symptoms are much worse as any pediatrician can tell you. It goes without saying that should you notice any of these symptoms, see your doctor and have appropriate tests done.

5. Treatment and prevention

As we do not see acute lead poisoning now as much as in the past, except sadly to say still in development countries and highly industrialized areas with lead emissions into the air, I like to emphasize the importance of prevention here.

a) If you absolutely must have make-up and/or lip sticks or lip gloss, at least go for the expensive, organic products. You owe it to yourself. However, having said that keep in mind that anything you put on your skin anywhere is absorbed to a certain percentage. So, why mess with your body's metabolism? I really question this. For your skin you can use a product called "Youth serum" from LifeExtension, where only a few drops will suffice to cover your face and neck with a thin film. Within a few seconds this is absorbed into the skin and it will stimulate your skin to grow where wrinkles are, so the wrinkles flatten out in time. Make-up conceals skin defects but this product restores your skin.

b) Keep in mind that skin appearance is hormone dependent; males need testosterone as they age and women need bioidentical progesterone. Some medical publications claim that progesterone would be cancer

producing. This is not true: it is progestin, a synthetic copy of progesterone that does this. Bioidentical progesterone in cosmetics is cancer preventing in women. It is advisable that men avoid skin contact with a woman who has applied such a product for at least two hours. Skin transfer of progesterone to men will block testosterone production in men! Worse still: if a manufacturer uses progestin (the synthetic version), the traces of it over a long period of time will act like xenoestrogens, which can cause breast cancer in the woman who uses such a product and through transfer can cause prostate cancer in a man.

c) If you insist on using chemicals on your skin, you may want to consider seeing a naturopathic physician who does intravenous chelation. Lab tests are available to assess the levels of heavy metals and toxins in your body. If the levels are creeping up, chelation treatments may be needed from time to time in people who have elevated lead levels in blood tests and/or urinary tests. Discuss this with your doctor. Removal of any accumulated mercury, lead, cadmium or other heavy metals is highly recommended. I have summarized detoxification methods in a blog entitled "Get rid of toxins safely"(see references).

Conclusion

In conclusion, I think that it has to be carefully considered, how much lipstick application is necessary. Next the choice of a high quality product is of utmost importance. Taking all the factors together, its constant use cannot be recommended, especially since there is not only lead present, which is a known health hazard. Beside lead there are many other chemicals that get absorbed, and their effects have not been adequately tested by the agencies.

Protection from radioactivity

Even though the Chernobyl catastrophe was bad enough, it appears now the 2011 Fukushima Daiichi nuclear power plant catastrophe was 7 to 10 times worse in terms of worldwide radioactive pollution. Even as late as Feb. 20, 2014 there was a new report of a further radioactive water spill into the Pacific Ocean.

It is important that you start thinking about preparing yourself to cope with radioactive pollution.

I will briefly review the history of several radiation disasters in various parts of the world and will mention how methods that help you to cop with radiation were fortuitously developed. Finally, I will summarize what you can do to reduce any damage to your health that is caused by radiation leaks.

History of the first nuclear bombs with radioactive fallout in 1945

On Aug. 9, 1945 the second atomic bomb was dropped on Nagasaki, Japan. Dr. Akizuki worked at the St. Francis Hospital (Uragami Daiichi Hospital), about one mile from the epicenter. He and a staff of 20 were serving at this hospital that looked after 70 tuberculosis patients.

Miraculously all of the staff and most of the patients survived because of a vegetarian diet, which consisted of uncontaminated brown rice, fermented foods, sea algae and vegetables. Dr. Akizuki did not allow sweets of any kind. Salt was allowed as the main condiment. Everybody was fed at least one helping of a soup with fermented soy and seaweed in it like wakame miso soup. Other investigators have confirmed that in a mouse model miso soup has radio protective effects.

The staff and the patients of another hospital also one mile from the epicenter of the second atomic bomb in

Nagasaki, Japan were not so lucky. Almost 100% of them died. They were not on the strict miso/seaweed diet without sugar and sweets.

The experience with Chernobyl

Perhaps the best way to start reviewing the Chernobyl disaster of April 26,1986 is by looking at how children fared who had been directly exposed to the radiation spill from this disaster. About 7 million people living in the nearby area were exposed to the highest radiation exposure ever recorded before. The children of this population have experienced a 2,400 % increase in thyroid cancers, a 100 % increase of cancers and leukemia and a 200% increase of breast cancer. There were about 800,000 men who risked their lives when working on containing the radiation spill. 25,000 of these men have died and 70,000 are disabled. 20% of the deaths (5000 men) were due to suicide. If you would like more details about the health consequences as a result of the Chernobyl disaster read the "Facts and figures about Chernobyl consequences" in the references. Questions and answers regarding the Chernobyl disaster can be found under "Q&A about Chernobyl" in the references.

The question is whether a similar accident could happen with any of the other nuclear power reactors. As one of the references explains such an accident can "only happen in a reactor operating with a Positive Temperature Effect combined with a Positive Steam Effect, and built without a containment structure to mitigate the potential atmospheric effects of a worst-case reactor accident." It goes on to say that only the reactor in Chernobyl was this type of a reactor, the RBMK series made by the former USSR. The reference explains further: "All other reactors for the production of electricity, including all those in America, operate on natural Negative Temperature and Negative Steam Effects, and are encased in air-tight multi-layered containments, the integrity of which rivals that of Egypt's pyramids." It ends with this rather strong statement: "This being understood, it is entirely correct to say that an accident like the one that occurred at Chernobyl in 1986, will never happen anywhere else." The same website reports in another section about the Fukushima disaster, without mentioning that this should not have happened. Nobody could have predicted the forces of nature, which was a double whammy of an earthquake of the magnitude 9 on the Richter scale, followed by a horrendous tsunami. This destroyed part of the nuclear power plant. From the literature it is not clear whether the government went through any major efforts to provide chelating agents, Prussian Blue and iodine salts to the affected population either in Chernobyl or in Fukushima to minimize the radiation effects from the radioactive emissions.

Part of the problem in Chernobyl was the fact that all of this happened behind the Iron Curtain, and at that time there was a news blackout. Information gradually improved only after 1989. In Japan the problem was severe denial and underreporting on behalf of the Japanese government.

Goiania accident involving radioactive cesium-137 in Brazil

On September 13, 1987 two fellows illegally entered an abandoned private radiation treatment hospital in Goiania in the Brazilian state of Goias where a radiation unit containing cesium-137 had been used for treating cancer patients. They stole the radiation head thinking that it might be valuable scrap metal that they could sell. They managed to sell it to a junkyard owner, Devair Ferreira.

Having a lack of insight that the radiation head would contain radioactive cesium-137, which was emanating ionizing radiation, Devair proceeded to probe for a precious metal with a screwdriver. As the details in the Wikipedia link show, shortly after a total of 112,000 people were screened for potential radiation exposure. There were 4 deaths including the junkyard owner's wife, and his 6-year old daughter. He himself survived the incident. 249 people were significantly contaminated with cesium-137, and 1000 people had received a dose twice the amount of the yearly background radiation. 20 patients developed radiation sickness and required treatment. The Brazilian authorities arranged treatments for patients who had proven contact with cesium-137 with 10 Grams of Prussian Blue daily, which reduced the effective radiation exposure by 70% as explained in the reference "Cesium-137, a deadly hazard". This was the reason for the relatively low mortality and disability rates from this serious radiation accident.

The Fukushima experience

Fast-forward to the latest disaster that has made it clear how an earthquake of the magnitude of 9 on the Richter scale followed by an enormous tsunami in combination could lead to the Fukushima disaster in Japan. Following the catastrophe on March 11, 2011 there have been several leaks of radioactive material into the ocean, which are described under the "Fukushima leak problems" reference.

Dr. John Apsley II pointed out that with the explosions in Fukushima there were also significant releases of radioactive pollution into the stratosphere that subsequently traveled around the globe. He has made it his ambition to help people minimize radiation exposure from nuclear accidents such as Fukushima.

The initial denial of the Japanese authorities caused a problem of assessing the true significance of the Fukushima incident.

As mentioned in the introduction to this blog there are still ongoing releases of radioactive material, which will eventually work their way into the oceans and into the atmosphere. Dr. Apsley II describes in detail in his book that there were 29 radioactive elements that were released into the air and into water, the main ones being Cesium-137 (and 134) Iodine-131, Plutonium-238 and 239, Strontium-89 and 90 and Uranium-234 and 238. As the body takes up these radioactive elements, they have different organ preferences and they metabolize differently so that each of them causes a certain disease pattern. Radioactive Iodine for instance causes thyroid disease and thyroid cancer, while radioactive Plutonium is causing leukemia, heart disease, lung and breast cancer, several childhood cancers and infant mortality. There is a wave of radioactive cesium-137 coming across the Pacific Ocean that has started to show up on the west coast of Alaska, Canada and the US mainland in early 2015 and will stay peaked until 2020 and beyond.

It is difficult to know the real concentration of the radioactivity in the water and in the radioactive rain over the US and Canada, as government agency measurements were kept hidden or were falsified. However the author comes to the conclusion in comparing various reference sources that the radiological leak and impact of the Fukushima crisis was and is about 7-fold to 10-fold bigger than that of Chernobyl.

Depending on what story you believe, the fear mongering or the more balanced reasoning arguing that there is enough water in the ocean to significantly dilute the amount of spilled radioactivity, you may or may not eat the sushi on the West coast as the news paper article "Is it safe to eat the sushi?" says under references.

With all the unclear information it is uncertain whether the local population made use of the simple method of chelation at home using miso soup and uncontaminated seaweed. One would hope so. But did they know that it is only effective in combination with a strict diet without sugar and starchy foods? The short-term damages are obvious now, but only the future will show how much illness, death and disability has come over the Japanese population due to this disaster.

Protection from radioactive fallout

This brings us to toxicity studies and simple ways of how to protect you from radiation in the environment. First, you need to know how radioactive materials can enter your body. Most nuclides (that is another name for radioactive compounds) enter the body through contaminated food via the gut where they are absorbed into your blood. You can inhale gases like gaseous radioactive lodine or Radon. Cesium, which has now leaked into the Pacific Ocean, can be absorbed through your skin when you walk barefoot on a beach that is contaminated with radioactive Cesium-137 containing ocean water. A link entitled "The Implications of The Massive Contamination of Japan With Radioactive Cesium" can be found under references. Cesium-137 has a half-life of 30 years, meaning that after 30 years it still emits 50% of today's gamma rays; and these are strong X-rays! The biological half-life of Cesium-137 in the body is 110 days. But we do not want this stuff in our bodies causing free radicals to destroy our body cells. So we need effective methods to remove radionuclides.

By reviewing the history above, we already have learnt of two effective ways to remove such radionuclides: Miso soup with seaweed in Nagasaki; and Prussian Blue in Brazil. Prussian Blue works on eliminating the radioactive Cesium-137 before it is absorbed from the gut into the blood. It disappears from the body with bowel movements and is also eliminated in the urine. However, it should

only be taken, when there is proven food contamination with Cesium-137 as it can seriously affect your potassium levels, which could cause serious side effects to your heart. A physician knowledgeable in the use of Prussian Blue can monitor your potassium levels and follow you along.

In comparison to that it is easy to implement dietary habits as was done in Nagasaki: miso soup and seaweed can be consumed without any side effects. So, why is it important to avoid sugar and starchy foods? The reason is that sugar oxidizes your cholesterol and any tissue it comes in contact with. It also causes the pancreas to overproduce insulin, which causes an inflammatory reaction. Cesium-137 also causes an extreme inflammation in your body, because of the free radicals that are released as the gamma radiation interacts with your body cells. Add to this a situation where there is a fire burning inside of your body, namely inflammation from sugar and starch consumption, and you have a recipe for disaster, comparing it to dumping gasoline into a fire. Inflammation is amplified and the radioactive Cesium-137 causes havoc in your system. You quench the fire when you do not eat sugar and starch and you give it an extra dousing by taking chelating agents, in this case miso soup with seaweed, which removes the radioactive Cesium-137. The successful outcome of Dr. Akizuki's treatments in his hospital in Nagasaki speaks volumes.

There are a number of other useful antioxidants like melatonin, vitamin C, and glutathione. Co-Q10 supports the mitochondria and protects cholesterol from being oxidized. But other substances are also useful. Cabbage contains isothiocyanates that will bind radionuclides before they are even absorbed from the gut. Edible clays, like calcium bentonite works in a similar fashion like Prussian Blue, but it also supplies extra calcium for the body. For further details consult Dr. Apsley's 2011 book, which contains a lot more details.

Conclusion

When I researched this topic the surprising twist for me was the fact that what is good for your heart, what prevents Alzheimer's disease and what helps you to live longer also helps you to cope with processing and eliminating radioactive pollutants. When we adopt a healthier lifestyle now, we are at the same time preparing ourselves to remove nuclear pollution from our bodies.

Update about the Fukushima fallout

I have written about the fallout from the Fukushima disaster in Japan in the previous section. It was projected that the levels of radiation found on the West coast of North America around 2015 would likely be high. It did take all that time for the water with the radioactive contamination to arrive on the Western shores of Canada and the US.

The predictions were based on the known water currents in the Pacific Ocean and the amount of radioactive pollutants released. With that data it was extrapolated what would happen in the future. At the time of writing this book the future is already here; we just heard about reports that the polluted water has arrived, but – surprise – the water radioactivity in early 2015 was much lower than predicted. Direct measurements of the radioactivity of the nuclear isotope composition in the water showed that the concentration is about 1000 times lower. We are lucky! We can swim in the ocean of the West Coast of the US and Canada and walk on the beach barefoot. The scientists who did the present calculations pointed out that swimming in the ocean for 6 hours for 7 days per week continuously for a period of one year would give you a radiation exposure 1000 times less than that of a dental X-ray. There is a Fukushima video under references that puts things into perspective. It appears that the dilution effect of the massive water mass of the Pacific Ocean was underestimated with the initial predictions.

I highly recommend watching the video clip. It sums up how the Fukushima disaster has affected marine life, but it also demonstrates that the West Coast of the US and Canada does not seem to be in danger of highly toxic levels of nuclear isotopes.

Why should we trust these measurements?

You may ask yourself: why should I trust these measurements? As pointed out in the previous section, there were a number of radioactive elements released into the atmosphere and into the Pacific Ocean. Cesium-137 and Cesium-134 are both part of the Fukushima incident. They have now been measured to be present in higher than previous concentrations at the coast of British Columbia. Cesium-134 has a much shorter half-life and can therefore only come from Fukushima. But Cesium-137 that has a half-life of 30 years was also increased to a higher than previous level because of the Fukushima disaster. Underwater nuclear weapons tests in the 1940's to early 1990 before the Comprehensive Test Ban Treaty was enacted caused the previous baseline of Cesium-137 levels in the ocean. Fortunately only about 25% to 30% of the original accumulated load of radioactivity was left before Fukushima added more Cesium-137. The other nucleotides Iodine-131, Plutonium-238 and 239, Strontium-89 and 90 and Uranium-234 and 238 are also helping scientists to sort out the contribution of radioactive pollution from Fukushima when compared to the baseline from underwater nuclear weapon tests before.

Why it matters what you eat

You may think that you are completely safe now that we have such good news about radiation associated with the Fukushima disaster. Not quite so. Any source of radiation, which includes traveling by plane, getting mammograms in women, getting CT scans, lung X-rays, dental X-rays etc. has an effect on your system. It causes an inflammatory response, which is made worse by sugar and starchy foods. Sugar and starchy foods have been known for some time to oxidize LDL cholesterol, which in turn causes inflammation in your arteries and travels through your whole body including your brain. Even Alzheimer's disease is an inflammatory brain disease, partially caused by overconsumption of sugar and starchy foods. Now add to this radioactivity exposure, which causes a strong inflammatory process in your body from free radicals that circulate in your blood. As a result the problem with the background radiation being a bit higher than what it used to be is adding to the oxidative stress from sugar and starchy foods causing even more inflammation within the body. We need to remember that the victims of Nagasaki, Japan were the ones that did not follow the dietary advice of Dr. Akizuki. He had ordered a strict vegetarian diet, which consisted of uncontaminated brown rice, fermented foods, sea algae and vegetables. Dr. Akizuki did not allow sweets of any kind. Salt was allowed as the main condiment. Everybody was fed at least one helping of a soup with fermented soy and seaweed in wakame miso soup.

It was this regimen that helped tone down inflammation in the body. It countered the negative effects of the radiation of the atom bomb.

Other causes of radiation

We are exposed to the leftover of 25% of the nuclear experiments from the nuclear bomb testing, the leftover radioactive Cesium-137 mentioned above. In addition background radiation from sunbursts and cosmic radiation have to be absorbed by our system. As the radiation fuels inflammation, we cannot afford to continue to indulge in sugar and starchy foods that lead to hyperinsulinism, inflammation and oxidation of LDL cholesterol. If we cast all caution to the wind, we will get degenerative diseases like arthritis, inflammation of the lining of the arteries leading to high blood pressure, heart attacks and strokes. Obesity and diabetes will also undermine our health. All of this leads to disabilities and premature deaths.

Conclusion

I am glad that the Fukushima news are a lot better than anticipated for the West Coast of the US and Canada. However, we should not forget that, like the burden of radiation, certain foods (sugar, high fructose corn syrup and starch) also cause inflammation in our system. We need to remember how effective Dr. Akizuki's diet was back in 1945 protecting those who were in immediate proximity to the atom bomb in Japan. Today we should consume a Mediterranean diet, which is also full of antioxidants, is thought to be anti-inflammatory and has been linked to slower aging.

We can also take antioxidant vitamins like vitamin C, glutathione, fish oil, vitamin D3 and others that will protect us from anything that oxidizes LDL cholesterol or produces free radicals. Common sense needs to prevail. Radiation is a burden that fuels inflammation in our bodies, but dietary measures can greatly contribute to keeping us out of trouble.

Chelation for detoxification - does it work?

Even though the Trial to Assess Chelation Therapy (TACT Study) has been published in March 2013, it still needs to make its way into the common public knowledge. The National Institute of Health was noticing an "alarming 68% increase" of chelation therapy between 2002 and 2007. These patients had problems with previous heart attacks and others had angina due to coronary artery disease, so they sought relief through intravenous chelation treatments. The purpose of the TACT study was to see whether chelation treatments with EDTA were safe and whether they would show any benefits when compared to a placebo group.

TACT study design

A total of 1708 patients were randomized into two groups, 869 treated with EDTA chelation therapy and 869 in treated with placebo infusions of normal saline/dextrose. Treatments were blinded (nobody knew what was given in the intravenous). 134 research sites in Canada and the US were involved in this trial including the Mayo Clinic. Patients had to be at least 50 years old, but the average age was 65 years. They had all a prior heart attack, but not less than 6 weeks before enrolment; on average they did have their heart attack 4.6 years before enrolment. Participants had to quit smoking at least 3 months before entering into the study and if they had revascularization procedures like a bypass surgery or stents, this had to be done more than 6 months in the past.

31% of the study population had diabetes. 83% had revascularization procedures done in the past. The majority of patients were taking heart medications (72% beta blockers, 73% statins to lower cholesterol and 84% aspirin to thin the blood).

65% completed 40 infusions, 76% completed at least 30 infusions.

The chelation infusion was the standard infusion usually used in chelation clinics, namely containing EDTA, the chelating agent, salts and vitamins as indicated in the Mayo clinic summary report. The follow-up period was for 4 years. There was a dropout rate of 30% for various reasons and 17% refused their consent to carry on in the study.

Results of the TACT study

Overall mortality in the chelation group was down 2.8% versus the placebo group. Heart attacks in the chelation group were down 19.5%; strokes down 20% and hospitalization rates were down 28.6% when compared to the values of the placebo group.

Diabetic patients (the subgroup of 31%) appear to have greater benefits from chelation treatments than the non-diabetic ones. The diabetic group benefitted by 39% with regard to risk reduction (strokes, heart attacks, mortality) versus the non-diabetic chelation group (only a 4% reduction).

Perhaps as important as the results of the effect of the chelation study versus the placebo group was the fact that the side-effect profile was indistinguishable between the two groups. This establishes for the first time that chelation therapy is safe and that it also has beneficial effects. It proves even for those who have their doubts that it works!

It is interesting to observe the reaction of health professionals, when the results of the TACT Study were announced at the 2012 American Heart Association meeting in Los Angeles. The majority of cardiologists did not believe the results that chelation was effective; instead they were looking for alternative explanations to explain the effect and suggested that this study needed to be repeated

again. In the meantime they begrudgingly admit that it was a well-designed study and was published in a reputable mainstream medical journal, the Journal of the American Medical Association, JAMA.

What are the benefits of chelation therapy?

Originally EDTA was used to treat children with lead poisoning in Germany. However, workers who were exposed to lead containing paints in various industries also were described to have improved significantly with EDTA chelation.

In the 1990's environmental concerns about heavy metal poisoning of the earth atmosphere came more into the forefront. A paper published in 2007 reports about heavy metal pollution and poisoning in detail.

A new concern for those who like organic food is the use of copper sulfate by organic food growers to spray against fungal and bacterial growth on crops, as copper sulfate is one of the 5 chemicals used in organic agriculture approved by the USDA. Those who consume organic foods may inadvertently expose themselves to copper in their system. This will reduce zinc levels as zinc naturally counterbalances the effects of elevated copper levels; zinc and copper must remain in balance. Normal zinc levels are needed for normal body function, particularly in males. A simple solution is to have the occasional chelation therapy treatment to remove the excess copper from the system.

As I have explained before, chelation therapy and several other methods can detoxify the body; I have written a blog about this entitled "Get rid of toxins safely". Pollution continues to play havoc with our system, and we need to consider taking steps to counteract that. I explained in the blog that we live in a toxic world and I mentioned several steps we can take to counteract damages including

chelation therapy. "Living in a toxic world" is a second blog that deals with detoxifying the body. Particularly heavy metals like lead; mercury, cadmium and copper will be reduced in the blood by intravenous EDTA chelation treatments and safely eliminated through bile and urine.

Conclusion

I felt that I should take some time explaining the carefully conducted TACT Study that was a randomized double blind, government sponsored study examining the effects of chelation treatments. It showed that there were significant improvements in terms of cardiovascular recovery, but it also showed that it was entirely non-toxic. Chelation should be done by an American College for Advancement in Medicine (ACAM) certified practitioner to ensure that you get the same chelation treatment as described in the TACT Study. People with heart conditions will need 30 to 40 treatments, usually 1 week apart or at the most two treatments per week, to improve. However, a person with a normal heart who considers detoxification will only need 10 treatments initially twice per week or weekly. One maintenance treatment could be done every three months. We all reside on the same planet and are exposed to ongoing pollution and food toxicity. Due to this reality the topic of chelation and detoxification is worth some serious consideration not only for patients with heart health issues, but also for those of us who want to live a healthy, long life without disabilities.

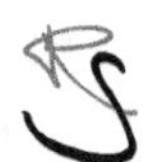

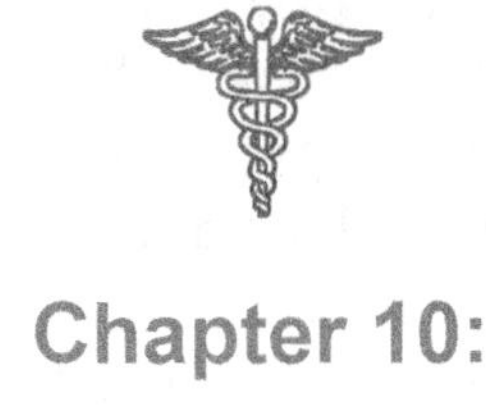

Chapter 10:

Reduce Impact from Cancer

Cancer is a disease that develops with the permanent metabolic changes at the end stage of chronic inflammation; at the same time the immune system is also broken down or severely compromised. Traditionally the medical profession has treated cancer like an enemy that has to be removed surgically, destroyed with radiotherapy or poisoned with chemical warfare, called chemotherapy. Never mind that there could be a spread of cancer cells with surgery, scarring and DNA damage to previously healthy cells due to radiotherapy and severe damage to the bone marrow with chemotherapy. This sounds very much like another case of "healing gone wrong". Hair falling out with chemo is considered to be only a temporary "minor side-effect". I have not met a patient who was happy about hair loss with chemotherapy.

Thankfully there are new approaches that have devloped treating cancer with more user-friendly methods.

In the first section I am asking the question whether cancer can be beaten. In the past it sounded more like a hollow promise or a cancer campaign slogan. But since Dr. Weber's successes in Germany with rainbow colored laser beams using photo laser therapy and utilizing various

photosensitizers, there have been amazing cures of metastasizing cancers that were thought to be impossible in the past. Cancer can be weakened, the immune system can be stimulated, and the result is that cure rates for various cancers can be increased significantly.

Next I am discussing lifestyle interventions that can prevent cancer. Removing sugar from our diet is a powerful cancer preventative. When it comes to skin cancer prevention, apart from sunscreens we will learn that we need to add prevention from the inside out: vitamin D3 and tropical fern (Polypodium Leucotomos).

Not long ago the Mayo Clinic has achieved an unconventional multiple myeloma cure with the measles vaccine. Multiple myeloma is a bone tumor that is otherwise very difficult to cure.

Back to cancer prevention: combine exercise with taking vitamin D3 and you will probably prevent half of all cancers, if not more.

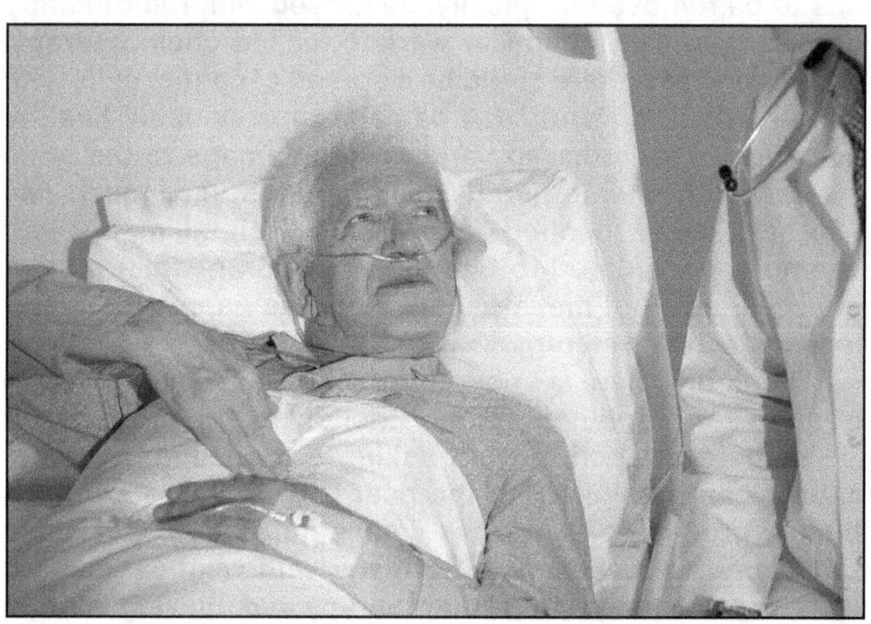

Can cancer be beaten?

For decades we have been indoctrinated that cancer can be beaten, but only marginal progress has been achieved with respect to effective cancer treatment modalities. Over time we almost have become accustomed to be negative about the answer to the question "can cancer be beaten?" But with the new developments that I will review below I like to propose that the answer is a resounding "yes". What has already been achieved needs to be further refined.

We know for a long time that there are distinct differences between the glycolytic cancer cell metabolism and the aerobic metabolism of normal cells due to the Warburg effect (see references).

In recent years the introduction of photochemical sensitizers followed by laser activation has made significant inroads regarding cancer treatment successes.

Animal experiments

Lithuanian researchers used a mouse model and reported about the use of several photosensitizers to treat Ehrlich ascites carcinoma in 2002. The most effective substance was Hypericin, which is derived from Hypericum perforatum, a plant also known as St. John's Wort. It showed the highest intracellular accumulation within the tumor cells, and the survival curves were the best with 25% cures after just one photodynamic treatment and a significant delay of mortality in the remainder of the animals. The control animals lived only 25 days on average, but the Hypericin pretreated and photodynamic therapy treated animals lived about 70 days with the cured ones still being tumor free at 120 days.

Experiments like these have taught the medical profession that the type of photosensitive agent (e.g. Hypericin) matters, particularly how well it is taken up by the tumor. The other important factor is the absorption pattern of the agent, as the choice of laser light will determine how good a match is achieved between the wavelength of the laser and the inherent peak excitation of the agent, also known as the absorption spectrum.

Laser treatment of a group of melanoma patients

In 2011 Dr. Weber described a report by Dr. M.A. Kaplan that was presented at the 2008 international laser conference in Helsinki. 76 patients with metastasizing melanomas were treated with Chlorin E6, a natural photo-sensitizer, and intravenous laser for activation. 45% had reduced pain and improved life quality, in 22% of the cases lymph nodes with metastases either disappeared or became smaller; in 33% the metastases stopped spreading for 6 to 12 months.

Photodynamic therapy of a patient with duodenal cancer and liver metastases

Dr. Michael Weber who is a specialist for internal medicine and the inventor of the Weber low-dose laser machine has treated cancer patients with photodynamic therapy (PDT) where his laser machine was used.

One such cancer case was a female patient with a duodenal cancer (Weber, to be published in 2015). She had a primary duodenal tumor removed in 2009 using the Whipple procedure. At that time 4 liver metastases were noted. She saw Dr. Weber in 2010 because of two rapidly emerging liver metastases. A first photodynamic therapy (PDT) was done in May 2010. She felt much better. In June 2010 a second PDT course was given. An MRI scan of the liver in July 2010 no longer showed any metastases. However, in December 2010 metastases reappeared in her liver, which were treated with 3 more sessions of PDT in

January of 2011. The metastases were still growing slowly. Dr. Weber decided to do a combination treatment with systemic PDT involving Chlorin E6, a photosensitizer and treating the metastases at the same time with interstitial laser therapy. Red light was used to stimulate the Chlorin E6. Miraculously the liver metastases became necrotic two weeks after this 20-minute treatment. Subsequently a surgical team from the University of Göttingen, Germany did a partial liver resection. At this point the patient appears stable and cancer free. This is a highly impressive achievement for an end-stage duodenal cancer case!

Photodynamic therapy of a group of inoperable prostate cancer patients

Dr. Weber treated 20 patients with prostate cancer with PDT between May and September 2014. 20% of them had a complete remission of their cancers. 35% experienced a partial remission; another 35% had no further tumor progression. In 10% the tumors progressed. These patients were given the following photosensitizers: 80 mg Chlorin E6, 10 mg Hypericin and 150 mg Curcumin intravenously. Three hours after the intravenous photosensitizers had been given photodynamic laser therapy (PDT) was administered through a transparent, permanent catheter that allowed admission of the laser instrument up to the level of the prostate. With this approach the low-dose laser light penetrated the entire prostate gland. Three frequencies were employed that corresponded to the absorption peaks of the three photosensitizers, red light (658 nm) to activate Chlorin E6, yellow light (589 nm) to activate Hypericin and blue light (405 nm) to activate Curcumin.

In addition to PDT patients also received an immunostimulator preparation, called Gc protein-derived macrophage activating factor (GcMAF). Finally, in order to take advantage of the minimal differences regarding poor oxygenation of cancer cells versus good oxygenation of normal tissues, intravenous oxygen was given with the oxygenation system of the German company Oxyven. This strengthened the normal tissue and weakened the cancer tissue.

The German researcher, Dr. von Ardenne did extensive research about the effects of oxygenation on healthy tissue versus cancer tissue. He postulated for instance that it would be possible to prevent cancer from metastasizing, if a person would exercise regularly while breathing oxygen through a mask. However, at this point this thought is not universally accepted and has not been proven in trials.

When all the effects are taken together, the photo-dynamic therapy with photosensitizers and specific laser frequencies, the immune therapy and the oxygen therapy, the above successes in treatment outcomes can be explained as a synergistic effect: cancer cells are dying off from the PDT, macrophage activating factor stimulates the immune system, and healing can start to occur.

Other end-stage cancer pilot studies

Dr. Weber reports about other pilot studies involving end stage breast cancer and pancreatic cancer (Weber, to be published in 2015).

Two cases of breast cancer with primary lesions measuring 3.5 cm or 5.0 cm were treated with Chlorin E6 and subsequent photodynamic laser therapy using the systemic and interstitial red laser of the Weber system. Within a few days tumor necrosis was visible and within 6 weeks after the PDT no tumor was present anymore in both cases.

Another case was an end stage pancreatic cancer in a 76-year-old man. This cancer was surgically removed in August of 2012. A few months later malignant ascites developed (cancer spread within the abdominal cavity). Chemotherapy with Gemzar had to be abandoned because of severe side effects. At this point PDT was started using Chlorin E6 twice with intraabdominal and intravenous red laser treatment. The patient also received a low-dose chemotherapy treatment with the pro-drug Xeloda, which gets converted into 5-fluoro-uracil (a standard chemotherapeutic agent). Using blue laser activation Xeloda becomes 100-times more powerful in destroying tumor cells. Only 3 months after this treatment the "incurable" pancreas cancer patient had been cured of his tumor and the malignant ascites. Initially the patient also had a secondary severe anemia that had to be treated with several blood transfusions before the PDT was started. Histology samples could no longer demonstrate presence of pancreatic tumor cells and the "intractable" anemia was cured as well. With conventional cancer therapies this patient would have been dead within 2 to 3 months.

Historic studies involving mega vitamin doses on end-stage cancer patients

Dr. Hoffer, the father of orthomolecular medicine, conducted an experiment on incurable cancer patients. Orthomolecular medicine is a branch of medicine that uses large doses of vitamins and minerals to rectify metabolic changes in various diseases. Dr. Hoffer treated 131 advanced cancer patients between 1976 and 1988 with a mixture of mega vitamins and minerals. This group taking the mega vitamins and minerals was the experimental group. There was also a control group that did not take any supplements. The results of this 9-year follow up study are depicted as an image in my blog http://www.askdrray.com/can-cancer-be-beaten/.

The Y-axis represents the % of survival (at the zero point of time 100 % of each group were alive); the X-axis shows the time of survival in years. The group of cancer patients taking mega vitamins is depicted with orange columns, the control group with blue columns. At 7 years of follow-up none of the controls survived, but 39% of the mega vitamin group cancer patients were still alive. On average there was an 8-year survival advantage of the mega vitamin group versus the control group (control group 28% survival at year 1 of follow-up, mega vitamin group 34% survival at year 9 of follow-up). The supplements consumed were as follows:

Vitamin C, 10,000 to 40,000 mg orally daily; vitamin B3 (niacin or niacinamide) 300 to 3,000 mg; vitamin B6 (pyridoxine) 200 to 300 mg; folic acid 1 to 30 mg; vitamin E succinate 400 to 1,200 IU; Coenzyme Q10 300 to 600 mg; selenium 200 to 1,000 micrograms daily; zinc 25 to 100 mg; calcium and magnesium supplement (2:1 ratio); mixed carotenoids as carrot juice; multivitamins and minerals.

Dr. Saul explains in his book that the Mayo Clinic did a study where they “duplicated” Dr. Hoffer’s study using only high doses of vitamin C, but failed to show any cancer fighting effect. However, they neglected to include all of the other cancer fighting supplements listed above. Vitamin C is an antioxidant, stimulates the immune system, but does not fight cancer by itself.

Conclusion

Cancer treatments are entering a new phase where with the help of multiple treatment modalities combined (PDT, immunostimulation, oxygen therapy and low-dose laser activated chemotherapy) it is now possible to cure many cancers that were untreatable in the past. The tunnel vision approach of conventional oncology with a combination of

surgery, chemotherapy and radiotherapy is obsolete for cases where cancer has metastasized. At this point the methods described here are still considered experimental. In Germany they have done phase 1 and phase 2 trials as indicated above. Large phase 3 trials will have to be performed involving various types of cancers through conventional cancer agencies. Intravenous and interstitial photodynamic therapy has the potential of replacing the traditional toxic ways to treat cancer. These new methods are effective with regard to both the primary tumor and metastases with hardly any side effects.

Please note:

Dr. Schilling has no commercial interest in Dr. Weber's low-dose laser system; the links provided in the reference section of this publication are merely there because of the newest information about low-dose laser photodynamic cancer therapy. Anybody who needs more information about the equipment or medical personnel wanting to buy the low-dose laser equipment can contact Jonathan Schwartz at this email: medicalmarvels@yahoo.com. Jonathan Schwartz is the sales representative for the Weber system in the US.

Lifestyle influences life expectancy

I have previously talked about telomeres, stem cells and lifestyle as themes. In this section you find summaries from three talks at the 22nd Annual World Congress on Anti-Aging Medicine In Las Vegas (Dec. 10-14, 2014) that dealt with telomere length and how nutrition can positively influence what our genes express. This ultimately determines how long we live. This is at the core of anti-aging medicine, and it is the reason why I dealt with it in some detail here.

1) Dr. Theodore Piliszek: "Personalized Genetics: Applying Genomics to General Health, Nutrition, and Lifestyle Modification"

Dr. Piliszek emphasized that everybody is different: metabolism is different from one person to the next. As a result of this, one needs to match the diet one recommends for a patient to that person's genetic make-up.

The Mediterranean diet has 20% protein, 35% fat, 45% carbs; here is the composition of other diets:

Low carb diet: 30% protein, 30% fat, 40% carbs

Low fat diet: 20-25% protein, 20-25% fat, 50-55% carbs

Balanced diet: 20% protein, 25% fat, 55% carbs

Snack only on low caloric foods; otherwise leptins react and make you hungry. A sweet tooth predisposes you to develop diabetes. Lactose intolerance is more common than previously thought. 30% of type II diabetics presently will develop dementia, and Alzheimer's is now often referred to as type III diabetes. With sugar being present in so many processed foods, the type II diabetes figure will likely jump to 60% in the future!

Methylation is very important for your well being. A quick reference about the methylation pathway explains methylation in simple terms without getting too much into biochemical nomenclature (see under references). Having said this, vitamin B2, B6, B12 are needed for this biochemical process and SAMe is also a supplement that supports methylation (SAMe).

If you do not have a longevity gene, you need to watch that you stick to organic food, stay active, and maybe add methylated folate and vitamin B12. Each patient should get a supplement list that is customized.

The health practitioner should ask the patient to keep a food diary for 1 week, which gives the doctor the nutritional profile including what the patient consumes in the way of drinks. Check vitamin D3 blood levels! Adequate levels of vitamin D3 are necessary for the musculoskeletal system and the immune system. Endurance training is important up to age 45. Beyond that age emphasis should be on isometric exercises (weight lifting or weight machines targeting different muscle groups).

Dr. Piliszek stated that the life expectancy in the US is falling behind many other countries. I did a quick Google check regarding life expectancy around the world as follows: US: 78.7 years; Canada: 81.2 years; France: 82.7, Italy: 82.9; Spain: 82.3; Portugal 80.37; Sweden: 81.7; Denmark: 80.05; Norway: 81.45; Germany: 80.89; Poland 76.8; Russia: 70.56. Seeing that the conference took place in the US, there is a lot of room for the US to improve habits with regard to food intake.

Dr. Piliszek stated that the normal range for hemoglobin A1C is skewed in the medical literature and the recommendations are too high; it should be: 3.8 to 4.9%.This is very important to know for diabetics and any caregiver who looks after diabetes patients, because if you are satisfied with a hemoglobin A1C of 6.0 as still being "normal", the diabetic patient dies prematurely of a heart attack or a stroke. Contrary to WebMD and the National Diabetes Information Clearinghouse (NDIC) recommendation it is important to take note: the new normal range for hemoglobin A1C is 3.8 to 4.9%! A patient whose hemoglobin A1C is 5.5 has diabetes and needs to be treated aggressively to prevent complications associated with diabetes.

2) George Rozakis, MD: "Nutrigenomics"

This talk focused on how one could use nutrition to heal when genetic errors are present in the metabolism.

This field is called “nutrigenomics”. It deals with using diet modifications and nutrients to change gene expression. Another way to express this is that with proper epigenetic changes and by using the right nutrients for a person with an inherited weakness, this measure can extend the life of this person. At the same time you need to avoid nutrients that would harm a person with a certain genetic weakness.

We all have inherited some minor or not so minor genetic errors in the genetic code. We are made up of 50 trillion cells with 30,000 genes and 23 pairs of chromosomes, so there are bound to be a few minor genetic code errors that make us more or less susceptible to develop disease. When we age our telomeres are shortening, making self-repair of many of our aging cells difficult, if not impossible.

Genes program our cells to run biochemical reactions within the cells. Correct methylation pathways are important for normal cell function. However, if there is a methylation defect, abnormalities set in and homocysteine accumulates.

With various enzyme defects you need to use appropriate supplements to normalize the metabolic defect. Vitamin B2, B6 and B12 supplementation will often stabilize methylation defects, and homocysteine levels return to normal. This is important as severe, familial cardiovascular disease can be postponed by several years or more just by using some supplements.

In a similar vein Dr. Rozakis mentioned that 92% of migraine sufferers have a defective methylation pathway involving histamine overproduction and they can be helped with a histamine-restricted diet.

Autism, ADHD (hyperactivity) and learning disabilities are other diseases where methylation pathway defects are present. Every patient with autism should be checked for methylation pathway defects, and appropriate supplements and diet restrictions can help in normalizing the child’s metabolic defects. DAN physicians, named for "defeat autism now", are well versed in this and should be consulted.

S-adenosylmethionine defects are another type of methylation defect, which is important in certain liver, colon and gastric cancers.

Dr. Rozakis went on to say that methylation defects lead to unbalances between T and B cells of the immune system and are important in autoimmune diseases like lupus or rheumatoid arthritis.

Methylation defects can also cause autoimmune thyroiditis and type 1 diabetes. They can also cause cardiac disease by raising homocysteine levels, which causes dysfunction of the lining of arteries and premature heart attacks.

Epigenetic factors can cause many different cancers through global methylation defects from vitamin B2, B6 and B12 deficiency. Hypomethylation is the most common DNA defect of cancer cells.

Mental illness is another area where epigenetic factors play an important role. Depression that responds only partially or not at all to SSRI's (antidepressants) often responds to L-methylfolate, a simple supplement from the health food store. Similar epigenetic approaches can be used to treat psychosis, schizophrenia, bipolar disorder and Alzheimer's disease.

With skin diseases it has come to light that atopic dermatitis, eczema, psoriasis, scleroderma and vitiligo are related to defects in methylation.

When we age, certain hormones are gradually missing, which leads to menopause and andropause. This leads to impaired cell function, elevated cholesterol, arthritis, constipation, depression, low sex drive, elevated blood pressure, insomnia, irritable bowel syndrome and fatigue. Replace the missing hormones with bioidentical ones and these symptoms normalize.

3) Dr. Al Sears: "Telo-Nutritioneering: The latest generation of telomere modulators".

The speaker pointed out that shortened telomeres are causing cells to behave like old cells. In the lab we can lengthen telomeres. Telomerase activated animals regrew their brains! In the human situation the goal is to find ways to preserve the length of our telomeres in all our key organs. Alternatively this can also be reached by inhibiting the breakdown of the enzyme telomerase, which will lead to a lengthening of telomeres. In his research Dr. Sears found at least 123 nutrients, vitamins and natural compounds that will elongate telomeres, often by stimulating telomerase.

Testing for critically short telomeres (HT Q-FISH method) is clinically more important than using average telomere length tests (Telomere testing). Dr. Sears said when a patient has been shown to have short telomeres and this patient is started on telomerase stimulating supplements, telomere lengthening can be documented within one month of starting the supplementation. Acetyl-L-carnitine and resveratrol are two substances that reliably elongate telomeres.

Vitamin C will significantly delay shortening of telomeres, which translates into delayed aging. In addition vitamin C has recently been shown to stimulate telomerase activity in certain stem cells. There is an herb, called Silymarin extract, which was found to increase telomerase activity threefold. N-acetyl cysteine is a building block for glutathione, a powerful anti-oxidant. In addition it has been shown to turn on the human telomerase gene. Other telomerase stimulators are green tea extract, ginkgo biloba, gamma tocotrienol (one of the components of the vitamin E group), vitamin D3 and folic acid.

Dr. Sears suggested that we should take the following supplements and vitamins for "telo-nutritioneering" with recommended dosages:

Acetyl L-carnitine: 1,000 mg daily; alpha tocopherol: 400 IU daily; folic acid: 2 mg to 5 mg daily; gamma tocotrienol: 20 mg minimum daily; ginkgo biloba: 40 mg to 80 mg daily (cycle every 4 to 6 weeks); green tea (EGCG): 50 mg daily; L-arginine: 500 mg to 1,000 mg daily; N-acetyl cysteine: 1,800 mg to 2,400 mg daily; resveratrol: 10 mg to 20 mg daily; silymarin: 200mg twice daily; vitamin C: 540 mg minimum daily; and vitamin D3: 2,000 IU daily.

Even if you are only taking 5 or 6 of these twelve telomerase boosters daily, you are doing well, particularly if you are also watching your lifestyle (regular exercise, not smoking, cutting out excessive alcohol intake and avoiding sugar).

Conclusion

This is only the beginning of rethinking epigenetic treatment approaches. For too long organized medicine has used a "cookie-cutter" approach of diagnosing and treating diseases. Now we are realizing that changes in hormones and shortening of telomeres with aging can cause inflammation and premature deaths. The future of medicine, which has already started, uses nutritional changes, vitamins and supplements, bioidentical hormone replacements and exercise to stabilize cell metabolism and postpone age-related diseases. In the context of the title of this book you may want to contrast this as "Healing Done Right" versus "Healing Gone Wrong".

Sugar can cause cancer

It has been known for a long time that cancer cells can survive without the ordinary aerobic pathways of energy production, called aerobic glycolysis. They can get energy from a metabolic pathway, called anaerobic glycolysis. But many attempts of designing a cancer therapy to exploit this difference have so far been unsuccessful.

The Mayo Clinic website says "it's a myth that people with cancer should not eat sugar" as the cancer would grow better with sugar. The following research questions whether this is really only a myth.

Sugar makes cancer grow faster (activates oncogenes) in fruit flies

In this study from the Icahn School of Medicine at Mount Sinai in New York City fruit flies were used as an animal model. You may ask, why fruit flies? We are not fruit flies, we are humans! As incredible as it sounds, on a cellular level our cell metabolism and the cell metabolism of fruit flies is identical. But the generation time of fruit flies is much shorter and results can be seen in days and weeks. To achieve the same results in human trials would take months and years. Also, researchers could breed a strain of fruit flies that was susceptible to develop tumors. When they were fed sugar, the fruit flies developed insulin resistance within a short time. This model was chosen by the researchers, as it is known for some time that in humans insulin resistance from diabetes, obesity, and other metabolic diseases leads to a higher risk of developing breast cancer, liver cancer, colon cancer and pancreatic cancer. The researchers wanted to sort out what the metabolic advantage of the cancer cells was due to these conditions.

The researchers found that the sugar from the diet was activating silent cancer causing genes, called "oncogenes" which in turn helped to promote insulin resistance and tumor development. Because of the insulin resistance sugar could not enter into the normal body cells, but the tumor was using up all of the sugar, which allowed the tumor cells to multiply at a rapid rate. The end result was that the sugar from the diet fed the cancer cells directly making them grow faster. Interestingly, when fruit flies that had developed tumors on a high sugar diet were switched to a high protein/low sugar diet, the tumors stopped growing and were contained.

In this fruit fly example the researchers were subsequently able to block cancer cell growth by special cancer suppressing drugs (acarbose, pyrvinium and an experimental drug AD81), which were given in combination. 90% of the flies given the triple-drug treatment survived to adulthood while control flies not treated with this regimen all died of their tumors.

Although this model was only done in fruit flies and one could question whether or not this was relevant to what is happening in human cancer patients, the following piece of research puts these doubts to rest.

Human breast cancer cell study in vitro

In January 2014 the American Society for Clinical Investigation published a collaborative study between the Lawrence Berkeley National Laboratory, Berkeley, California, CA and the Hokkaido University Graduate School of Medicine, Japan, which used human breast cells in tissue culture showing that sugar could cause breast cancer.

The original papers of this US/Japanese research team are quite technical. Under references you can find a reference, which I termed "Sugar causes cancer". The researchers used a simple tissue culture model where they could observe tumor growth in cell cultures under the microscope using a gel where the breast tissue samples were placed side by side with normal breast cells that served as controls; this is called a three-dimensional cancer model. The cell cultures of both normal cells and

malignant cells were obtained from the same reduction mammoplasty tissue samples from patients. This way the cell cultures mimicked a situation as close to the reality of what is going on in a woman's body when breast cancer develops.

The normal breast epithelial cells were seen in culture to get organized as a roundish cell formation a so-called "acinus formation", while the cancer cells were growing as irregular cell clumps. This visual effect was reproducible and is depicted in the paper, which under references I called "sugar promotes oncogenesis". With high sugar concentrations in the growth medium breast cancer cells multiplied at a faster rate, not so the normal cells. In addition some normal cells underwent a transformation into abnormal and cancerous cell types. On the other hand, when sugar concentrations were severely restricted, morphological changes took place where cancer cells slowed down their growth or stagnated while some of them even changed into the normal acinus cell formation. Using various known oncogene stabilizers the investigators could show that the same effect was noted as with the low sugar concentration in the growth medium.

The investigators tested whether other cell lines of breast cancer would show similar results as sugar feeding or restriction. They were able to show that high sugar feeding activated cancer cells, no matter where the cancer cell lines originated from. The authors discussed that metformin, which is known to control the metabolism in diabetic patients and lowers blood sugar levels, has also been shown to calm down growth of cancer, which is due to stopping oncogene stimulation. It can improve the survival rates of diabetic patients with many different cancer types. Those who take metformin can also reduce the risk of developing cancer.

Other investigators have shown in mouse experiments that low carb diets achieved an impressive lowering of cancer rates.

Human evidence for cancer causation and cancer prevention

Several clinical studies indicate that there is a higher cancer rate in diabetics where insulin resistance can lead to activation of cancer producing genes, called oncogenes causing various cancers. There is a discussion of colorectal cancer and pancreatic cancer showing a clear relationship to diabetes and insulin resistance. High glycemic foods such as sugar and starchy foods were associated with breast cancer, colorectal cancer and endometrial cancer. The majority of trials showed this association, although not all. The more obese patients were, the more pronounced the insulin resistance was, and the more the relationship to these cancers became apparent. A diet that is high in starchy foods like potatoes, rice and bread is causing pancreatic cancer as was shown by researchers at the Dana-Faber Cancer Institute, Brigham and Women's Hospital and Harvard School of Public Health. You can find their reference under the heading "high starch linked to cancer". In a Harvard study high glycemic diets have shown to cause colorectal cancer, diabetes and being overweight. The Standard North American Diet (SAD) is a pathway to many chronic illnesses due to its high load in refined carbs. Ironically the abbreviation for it is "SAD", which in my opinion reflects adequately its sad influence on health and well being. We know now that sugar and starchy foods lead to insulin overproduction, which in turn causes the metabolic syndrome, also known as "insulin resistance". This causes the immune system to weaken and fat to be deposited as visceral fat in the stomach area. Visceral fat is metabolically very active as it secretes cytokines like tumor necrosis factor alpha (TNF alpha), COX-2 enzymes and others. Insulin and growth factors from the visceral fat gang up together with the elevated blood sugar, which activates tumor-producing genes, called oncogenes, to cause cancer.

While cancer rates are higher in patients with insulin resistance, they were lower in patients who did have normal insulin levels. It is important to concentrate your efforts on normalizing weight, which will normalize insulin sensibility and avoid the development of cancer. Sugar avoidance and avoidance of cereals and starchy foods will help you achieve this goal.

Conclusion

Although the idea that sugar could cause cancer has been around since 1924 when Dr. Warburg suggested it first, it has taken up to now to be proven in animals and humans.

The purpose of this section was to show how there is a connection between the consumption of sugar and starchy foods and various cancers in man. Animal experiments are useful in suggesting these connections, but many clinical trials including the Women's Health Initiative in 2002 have shown that these findings are also true in humans. It is insulin resistance due to sugar and starch overconsumption that is causing cancer.

We are now in a position to know why people who consume a low carb diet, develop less cancer than people who consume a high carb diet. I have followed such a low carb diet (also known as low-glycemic index food diet) since 2001 and find it easy to follow. However, I do not dispute that it takes some discipline to change the old way of eating to the new way. The benefits are definitely worth it: you are

feeling well and energetic and you actively contribute to staying well as you age.

Sunburn prevention

Much has been written about sunburn prevention. The thinking behind this is that perhaps we could prevent skin cancer and melanoma development, if we would block ultraviolet rays from the sun or from tanning booths and stop those rays from irritating our skin.

So far the theory. Now the truth. Here are some facts to think about.

1. Skin cancer

It is sobering that statistics of skin cancer frequency show that despite more awareness of the importance of skin protection with sunscreen lotions and creams, skin cancer rates have steadily increased. Behind this paradox is the fact that vitamin D3 production in the skin is blocked from sun exposure and the person is not getting the cancer protecting effect of vitamin D3.

Low vitamin D3 levels (measured as 25-hydroxy vitamin D levels) are not only associated with skin cancer, but also with breast cancer, and breast cancer will be reduced to 50% of control groups, if patients are treated with high vitamin D3 supplements. There are many other cancers that respond to exposure to sunlight or to supplementation with vitamin D3.

2. We need to know about infrared rays and the ultraviolet exposure

The ultraviolet radiation of sunlight has been extensively studied. There are UVA rays that range from 315 to 400 nanometers. They make up about 95% of the sunlight and

penetrate deeper into the skin (the dermis level) leading to more severe skin damage, producing aged looking skin. UVB rays (5% of sunlight) contain wavelength measuring between 280 and 325 nanometers affecting the most superficial layer of the skin, the epidermis. These rays cause sunburns. Both UVA and UVB are strongest around midday. The sun also produces UVC rays (wave length 180 to 280 nanometers), which are completely absorbed by the ozone layer and are not of importance unless you live under an ozone hole.

Next there is IR (infrared radiation), which has only recently been detected to be of health concern. IR rays range from 760 nanometers to 1 million nanometers (=1 millimeter). It causes skin photoaging and damage. Most of IR is in the lower range (between 760 and 1,440 nanometers); the total amount of IR rays that reach the skin is massive compared to the UV light and 50% of these rays reach deep into the skin to the level of the dermis.

3. Filtering out the damaging rays

Armed with the above knowledge we can now talk about sunscreen lotions and sunscreen creams. Traditional sunscreen lotions and creams have been directed against both shortwave (UVB) and longwave (UVA) rays of the sun. UVB blockers prevent damage to the surface of the skin (epidermis level), UVA blockers prevent damage to the deeper dermis. It is in your interest to buy a sun-blocking agent that blocks both of these rays. You have to read labels!

However, both of these blockers, which means all of the traditional sunscreen agents, will not block IR waves (infrared radiation), which causes most of the wrinkles, age-related skin changes and skin DNA damage, which can eventually also result in skin cancer.

4. Vitamin D3 deficiency because of sunscreen applications

We know that sunscreen agents lead to blocking of vitamin D synthesis in the skin; so it is prudent to take vitamin D3 5,000 to 10,000 IU per day and have your health care provider order 25-hydroxy vitamin D blood levels from time to time. Aim for a blood level of 50 to 80 ng/ml. There is no danger of overdosing vitamin D3. That story about overdosing of vitamins is coming from vitamin A overdosing. There is a ceiling not to be exceeded due to liver toxicity regarding vitamin A overdosing, but not so for vitamin D3. Vitamin D3 protects not only from skin cancer, but also from other cancers. For more on vitamin D3 you may want to read my blog on the superpowers of vitamin D3 (see references).

5. Whole body protection from the inside

There are two approaches to using systemic natural extracts. One component is from a tropical fern (Polypodium leucotomos) and another one from blood oranges that can both repair sun damaged skin and prevent sunburn. The effective substances are administered orally.

This fern extract has been tested in smaller clinical trials and was found to have a 70% to 75% efficacy in blocking all sunrays from the inside out.

In a small trial patients were exposed to UVB light after preparation with red orange extract and a 35% reduction of sun burn was found within 15 days when compared to controls.

There is a possibility now to take one capsule of tropical fern extract mixed with red orange extract and combine this with traditional sunscreen agents to have optimal sun protection.

One trial involved a group of patients with polymorphous light eruption, meaning that these patients were born with extreme sun sensitivity. They reported an 80% improvement with this oral fern extract treatment in these patients.

6. Final recommendations for sunburn prevention

Although some of the advice of WebMD on sun protection is useful, it neglects to recommend to supplement with vitamin D3 because of the sunscreen action. It also does not mention the IR waves of the sun that do most of the damage and that only get prevented by staying out of the midday sun or by taking the oral sunscreen pill consisting of tropical fern extract and red orange extract.

My recommendation, provided that you are not allergic to ferns, is to consider taking the oral pill when you know you will be exposed to a lot of sunlight. As far as I know it is currently only available from LifeExtension as "enhanced fern block with red orange complex". It helps to block the entire wavelength of the sunrays. This will repair some of the skin damage that has already been done. Follow the WebMD link under references as well with regard to the sunscreen lotions/creams. Also stay out of the noon sun between 11 AM and 2 PM and take your vitamin D3 in the high dose range as discussed above to preserve optimal resistance against all kinds of cancers including skin cancer.

Conclusion

Prior to writing this section I was quite bewildered how misleading a lot of the literature is regarding the prevention of sunburns, particularly by assuming that all you had to do was to block UVB and UVA rays.

I attempted to explain why this is an oversimplification, and the skin cancer statistics clearly show that sunscreen blockers alone are not stopping skin cancer. We do need a combination of the following:

1. Staying out of the noon sun (11AM to 2PM).

2. Using clothing and wide sun hats to keep the sun out of our faces.

3. Use the traditional sunscreen agents. Reapply, if necessary.

4. Using an oral sunscreen agent that blocks infrared rays as discussed under point 5 and 6 above.

5. Using vitamin D3 in high doses as discussed under point 4 above for cancer prevention.

With this in mind, enjoy the sun!

When medical tradition fails - the unconventional cancer cure

Mayo Clinic physicians were desperate when two patients with end stage multiple myeloma, a vicious bone tumor, did not respond to chemotherapy; so they tried something unconventional: high doses of the measles vaccine in an attempt to stimulate the immune system.

Canadian researchers had reported in 2011 that oncolytic viruses created by genetically modifying small-pox vaccine virus, would enter tumor cells of patients but not damage normal cells. A high percentage of the end stage patients responded with tumor regression. Now the Mayo Clinic clinicians used high doses of a modified measles

vaccine to attack the multiple myeloma cells of two end stage patients, and it worked on at least one patient who is cancer free after a recheck of the bone marrow 6 months later. The other patient experienced a significant remission, something not heard of in an incurable end-stage condition. You can find the story in the media under the heading "Measles vaccine cures cancer" under references. This research is a new beginning for cancer researchers, as in the past the general thinking was that something as bad as cancer must be fought with something strong and toxic to get rid of the cancer cells. The emphasis was on "fighting the cancer cell". Now the emphasis is on "outsmarting the cancer cell".

With the modified measles vaccine the premise was to stimulate the immune system, which will fight the cancer much better. As a past cancer researcher I would say that it is about time to take this new approach as the old approach of attacking the cancer cell like an enemy with radiation and chemotherapy did not work too well. The new thinking is: why not stimulate the immune system to such an extent that it becomes newly activated, but to such a degree that there is no chance for the cancer cells to fight back. I searched the recent literature on PubMed regarding this topic and came across several other interesting human clinical trials. They are all smaller, but very encouraging. Here is a brief summary of what I found. You find all of the links under references in the back of the book.

***1. Prostate cancer vaccines:* In this 2014 article a review of the use of various vaccines with dendritic cells, viruses, or DNA are described directed against the prostate-specific antigen on the surface of prostate cancer cells.**

***2. Pancreatic cancer vaccines:* This cancer is very difficult to detect in the early stages, and as a result the**

outlook for chemotherapy or radiotherapy is extremely poor. Several approaches have been tried to use as an alternative. Immunotherapy is an option and the Mayo clinic researchers have already announced that the measles vaccine approach will likely be applicable to pancreatic cancer treatment as well in the near future. However, other clinical trials are on the way as was described in a paper dated 2013 to use other vaccination procedures.

3. Cervical cancer: The HPV (human papilloma virus) vaccine is targeting patients exposed to the high-risk HPV16 strain most often causing cervical cancer. It has been fast-tracked, and there are not only positive responses. At this point I cannot blame anybody who is guarded about the vaccine and possible side effects. On top of it, in 2013 researchers have described a phenomenon called "HPV immune escape", as some vaccinated women still developed cervical cancer. As a result a group of researchers are investigating how the vaccine could be improved by finding out how the immune system is being tricked in these cases by the HPV virus to bypass the antibodies of the vaccine. We are not looking at the final version of a completed vaccine yet!

4. Brain tumors (glioblastoma multiforme): This deadly brain tumor has a survival rate of only 15 months with conventional combination therapy. However, new anti-tumor vaccines are being tested in clinical trials as described in a paper in 2013, which already have shown much less toxicity than conventional therapies and they have longer survival times when compared to conventional therapy.

5. Melanoma treated with special vaccine: In the early 1970's the anti tuberculosis vaccine BCG was used to find that about 25% of patients had long-term survival advantages with this adjuvant treatment (original paper 1974). Recently several smaller clinical trials involving end stage melanoma patients utilizing various vaccines showed encouraging results with tumor regressions. Melanoma is a particularly vicious pigmented skin tumor. And yet, when messenger RNA (mRNA) was combined with dendritic cells and made into a vaccine, the antigen presenting T-cells that previously did not react against the melanoma tumor suddenly became very active destroying the tumors. This was published in 2014. This line of immune treatment is very promising and clinical trials continue to go on.

6. Another multiple myeloma treatment approach: Apart from the measles vaccine approach mentioned at the beginning of this blog, there is another approach that is being pursued at the Ohio State University Comprehensive Cancer Center and was published in 2014. Immune cells of patients with multiple myeloma are being modified in tissue culture to be more aggressive against a CS1 marker that is expressed on the surface of 95% of multiple myeloma cells in patients with this deadly cancer. The modified T cells are grown in culture and subsequently re-injected into the patients. In mice this research team found that 100% of animals treated with these CS1 activated T lymphocytes were alive at 44 days after treatment was started versus only 29% and 17% of two control groups. A phase I clinical trial on patients is coming up soon.

Conclusion

The encouraging news is that several of the clinical trials on humans seem to be showing breakthroughs with better survivals than in the past. In addition it is also encouraging to see that these new treatment modalities are non-toxic treatments, which compare very favorably with traditional chemotherapy and radiotherapy methods. Also, there is some recognition among cancer researchers that although mice or other animal species may be a good first screening method, the ultimate goal is to treat human patients. The treatment has to work for people, not just for a cage full of rodents! This means that cancer researchers need to concentrate on human cell lines and work with cancer patients. It will be interesting to see the outcome of these trials and new approaches; hopefully we will see better survival rates for cancer patients in the near future.

Vitamin D3 has super powers

Originally, when vitamin D was found to be the missing ingredient in preventing rickets in growing children the recommended daily allowance (RDA) to prevent rickets was found to be 400 IU of vitamin D3. The active metabolite of vitamin D has been identified as vitamin D3 for which the body has receptors on all vital organs such as the heart, brain, bones, kidneys, and liver. In recent years new insights have been gained as it turns out that the RDA's were set much too low for many diseases that can develop when vitamin D intake is too low, particularly in the aging population. Higher doses of vitamin D3 in the range of 800 to 1000 IU per day have been shown to prevent osteoporosis, falls and fractures in older adults and in nursing home populations. But the immune system of everyone is dependent on higher doses of vitamin D3. From Dec. 12 to 15, 2013, I attended an A4M conference in Las Vegas where Dr. Eisenstein reviewed in a lecture the latest on vitamin D3. It is now known that 2/3 of the US population is deficient for vitamin D as measured by blood tests. Their levels were less than 25 ng/ml. The standard test is the 25-hydroxy vitamin D level - abbreviated as 25(OH)D level. It is now known that you require at least a level of more than 40 to 60 ng/ml of 25(OH)D as measured in the US, which translates to more than 100 to 150 nmol/L measured in metric units in other countries, to prevent cancer. In the meantime (in 2015) the recommendation is to aim for a 25-hydroxy vitamin D level of 80 to 100 ng/ml. Toxic levels are only thought to occur above 200 ng/ml. For practical purposes a 25-hydroxy vitamin D level of between 50 to 80 ng/ml is adequate for most people. You should have this test done from time to time through your physician as absorption of vitamin D3 varies widely from person to person and you want to know how much vitamin D3 you need to take every day as a supplement to reach adequate blood levels to prevent cancer.

Metabolism of vitamin D3

90% of the vitamin D3 that we need comes from exposure to sunlight, which transforms a cholesterol metabolite (7-dehydrocholesterol) into the vitamin D precursor (vitamin D3 or cholecalciferol). This is what we absorb from naturally occurring fish oil and oily fish, but otherwise this does not naturally occur in foodstuffs. Dr. Eisenstein pointed out that it is well known that people living north of the 37th degree latitude lack vitamin D3 because of a lack of sun exposure, particularly in the winter season. People south of the 37th degree latitude have enough sun exposure, but wherever you live, it is advisable to have your vitamin D3 level measured as the 25(OH)D level, also because people absorb vitamin D differently. If you do not eat enough fish or fish oil, the levels likely are too low as is the case for 2/3 of the US population. Vitamin D3 supplements will have to be taken by those whose levels are too low. Vitamin D3 is further metabolized by the liver and then by the kidneys into the active vitamin D compound, called 1,25(OH)2D3, which is called “calcitriol”. The main effect of calcitriol is to absorb calcium and phosphate from the intestine into the blood stream. Together with vitamin K2, as explained previously, these minerals are then taken up by the bone to prevent osteoporosis or rickets in the growing child. What has not been known for a long time is that vitamin D3 is also necessary for normal cell metabolism by most of your body cells, but particularly by the vital organs like the brain, the heart, the kidneys, the liver, the immune system and the bone. However, doses of 5000 IU to 10,000 IU of vitamin D3 capsules per day are required for optimal vitamin D3 health. This will lead to levels of below 200 ng/ml of 25(OH) D levels, which have been proven to be safe. According to Dr. Eisenstein no toxicity has been found below 30,000 IU of vitamin D3 per day, but based on other authors a dose of 10,000IU should be adequate for most people.

I like to mention here that not every doctor agrees with Dr. Eisenstein that such large doses of vitamin D3 are necessary for prevention. The consensus in 2016 is that 25 hydroxy vitamin D levels of between 50 and 80 ng/ml as mentioned above are more reasonable as a normal target to prevent cancer.

Strangely enough colored people also have to take vitamin D3 supplements as the higher melanin pigment in the skin filters out UV light so effectively that their 25(OH)D level can be low. Always err on the cautious side and have your 25 hydroxy vitamin D blood level taken.

Vitamin D3 has a characteristic stereotactic configuration called a cis-triene structure, which allows it to bind free radicals and function as an antioxidant.

What are some of the clinical effects of vitamin D3?

1. Vitamin D3 has diverse effects on organ systems as Dr. Eisenstein summarized: vitamin D3 lifts depression and has been found to be of particular value for drug resistant depression. Take 5000 to 10,000 IU of vitamin D3 per day.

2. Muscle power increases with vitamin D3, particularly in those who work out regularly.

3. Many fertility clinics pay attention to vitamin D3 levels, as the higher the blood levels of vitamin D3 in a man, the faster this sperm cells move! And the more vitamin D3 the female has available in her body, the better she ovulates. The end result is a higher pregnancy success rate when both partners take 5000 to 10,000 IU of vitamin D3 per day.

4. Also, if a woman takes vitamin D3 during her pregnancy, the first set of teeth in the offspring will have fewer cavities.

5. Brain development in autistic children is much improved with vitamin D3 in higher doses. This needs to be combined with detoxification methods and supervised by one of the DAN physicians , the "defeat autism now" doctors.

6.Chronic pain typically improves when vitamin D3 deficiency is treated with vitamin D3 supplementation in patients with chronic pain. When patients with chronic pain are checked for 25 hydroxy vitamin D levels, vitamin D3 deficiency is often found.

7. To prevent flus and colds and other infectious diseases, take higher doses of vitamin D3. When you come down with a flu, it is safe to increase your daily vitamin D3 intake to 30,000 IU of vitamin D3 for a few days until your symptoms improve, then resume your maintenance dose of 5000 IU to 10,000 IU per day. In some years the type A, subtype H1N1 – also known as the swine flu was found to be the common type of influenza. Children should get 50% of the dose regimen detailed for adults when they develop a flu (for children: 15,000 IU for three to five days, with

tapering to a maintenance dose of 2500 to 5000 IU until blood levels of 25(OH)D are available). Under references you can find a website of Dr. Cannell where he discusses vitamin D3 dosages as well.

8. Asthmatic patients do better with vitamin D3 supplements requiring less maintenance anti-asthmatic medicine keeping them balanced with regard to their airways.

9. Chronic low vitamin D3 levels cause brain damage including Alzheimer's disease. In this context it is important to know that the enzymatic conversion in the liver and kidneys slows down as we age, requiring higher doses of vitamin D3 in older patients. This may have been the reason for the confusion about relatively low doses of 400 IU of vitamin D3 preventing rickets in children versus the need of vitamin D3 in middle aged and older patients where much higher doses are required as already explained. The target blood level of 25 hydroxy vitamin D is the same in children and adults: 50 to 80 ng/ml.

10. High blood pressure is linked to vitamin D3 deficiency and it blood pressure is easier to manage with medication when vitamin D3 levels are normalized.

11. Live longer with vitamin D3: How is this possible, you might ask: the answer has been found in the telomeres of the chromosomes, the shoelace like structures at the end of the DNA strand of each cell. Vitamin D3 lengthens the telomeres and promotes telomere repair; this is associated with a longer life span. Centenarians have longer telomeres. You can measure telomere length, but it is a pricey test, which is certainly not affordable for everyone, contrary to supplementation with vitamin D3 that is affordable for everyone and should be taken regularly!

12. As already indicated, vitamin D3 strengthens the immune system, but it also modulates the inflammatory response from muscle damage, so athletes can perform better. Patients with multiple sclerosis will improve as it slows down the inflammatory process. But other inflammatory diseases like arthritis, inflammatory bowel disease and even cancer will respond favorably to higher doses of vitamin D3. A necessary dosage can be 20,000 to 30,000 IU of vitamin D3 in these cases. This is information that has not yet percolated into mainstream medicine, but will do so in the next few years. At least one should hope so. Sometimes change can take decades.

13. Higher percentages of cardiovascular disease are found in patients who have lower than 15 ng/ml 25-Hydroxy vitamin D levels in their blood meaning that vitamin D3 supplementation prevents heart disease.

What are toxic vitamin D levels?

What is known about the safety of vitamin D3, particularly the higher vitamin D3 doses? First, it is wise to have your 25(OH)D blood levels taken from time to time. If any of these levels exceed 200 ng/ml it would be prudent to reduce the vitamin D dose or stop supplementation for a while. Otherwise it has been difficult to establish a toxic range.

There are claims that 40,000 IU of vitamin D3 or more would lead to toxic levels where the blood calcium levels would be increased, which can be measured as hypercalcemia. However, another study done in 2007 showed in MS patients that took 40,000 IU per day and that led to a blood level of 400 ng/ml of 25(OH)D did not lead to increased calcium levels and did not lead to hypercalciuria , which means too much calcium in the urine. So, all of the papers that either indicated to the public that it would be unsafe or unnecessary to take vitamin D3 seem to have other agendas than communicating the truth. Had it been true that calcium would be released from the bones or calcium was absorbed too much from the gut, this would have caused calcification of the bones, soft tissues, heart and kidneys. Also, kidney stones would have developed. However, a low calcium diet combined with corticosteroid drugs usually leads to a full recovery within a month. It is interesting that all of the dire predictions regarding toxic vitamin D3 levels did not materialize. You can read about this on another website discussing vitamin D3 dosing, one of them being WebMD: the truth about vitamin D.

I talked to a participant of the conference who has a fellowship degree of the A4M. I asked him what was really known about vitamin D3 toxicity. He told me that there has been an unintentional overdose where a compounding pharmacy made a mistake, so that a patient accidentally received a dosage of 500,000 Units of vitamin D3 per day for a full three months, before the mistake was uncovered. The patient felt sluggish, but did not have any other symptoms. He was told to stop the vitamin D3 compound. He had an uneventful recovery with no detrimental effects. At this point no overdose of vitamin D3 has been firmly established, but 200 ng/ml of 25-hydroxy vitamin D is the consensus value for the upper limit, beyond which toxicity could occur.

Conclusion

Vitamin D3 is a vital supplement that has been shown to prevent not only rickets in children, but also depression, MS, infections and even many cancers. As usual there will be many critiques that doubt the validity of the above statements, and negative rumors tend to linger for years. Nevertheless research has proven the benefits beyond any

doubt. Also after years where the recommended dosage of Vitamin D3 has been minimal, this vitamin has been found to be necessary in a higher dosage to give us its health benefits.

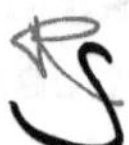

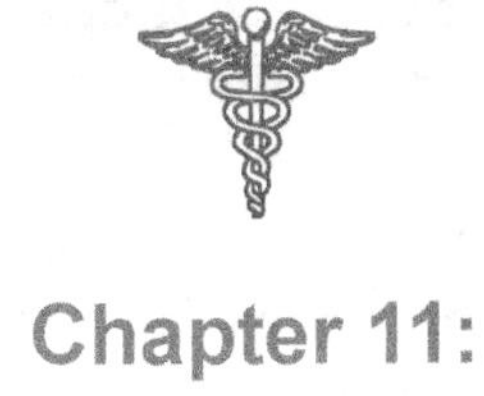

Chapter 11:

Stable Hormones Key to Health

As already mentioned earlier we are losing hormones, as we get older. With melatonin this starts happening after the age of 20, with DHEA and growth hormone after you are in your mid thirties. The big sexual hormone changes take place when we enter menopause or andropause, which is the male equivalent of menopause. Often more insidious is burnout, which is due to various degrees of adrenal gland insufficiency. Grumpiness in older men has been associated with a higher death rate; research found out that grumpiness is just another symptom of testosterone deficiency. The vital organs of a man need stimulation by testosterone.

Menopause

In men andropause, the equivalent of menopause is easy to spot and treat. With them it is about a lack of testosterone, which is confirmed with a blood test and treated with testosterone until the blood level comes back to normal and the symptoms disappear. Grumpiness is just one symptom. Often men notice lack of drive and a loss of erections and sex drive.

In women symptoms of menopause are more subtle, but more profound when they have them fully developed. Unfortunately there is a lot of misinformation out there, which includes communications from the media. As a result of this many women do not get treatment that would turn their lives around and make the next phase of life more livable. To my way of thinking this is simply not acceptable in a time when help is readily available. Read what I am writing here first and discuss this with your gynecologist or primary care provider. If you notice that there is a prejudice towards using synthetic hormones, go for a second opinion from a naturopathic physician. I will explain why later.

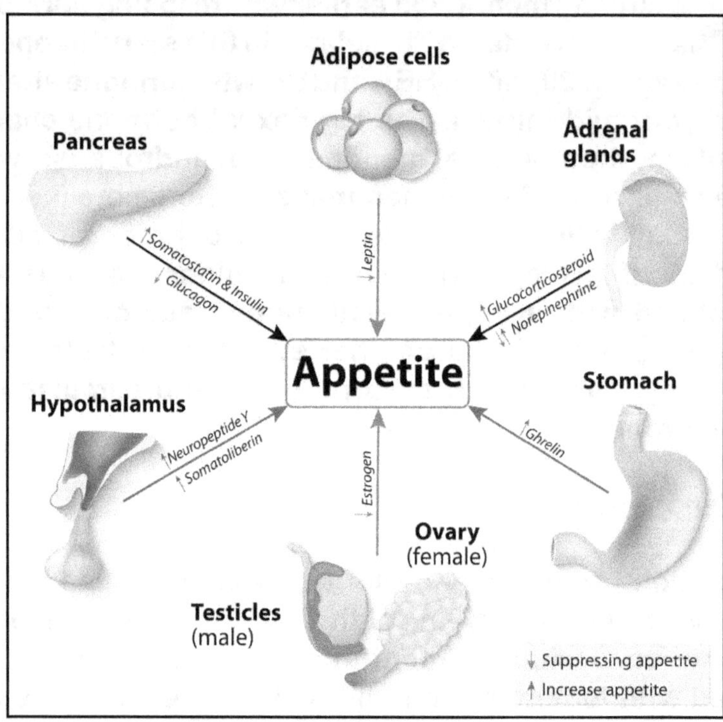

Confusion from the Women's' Health initiative in 2002

A discussion about menopause and hormone replacement therapy (HRT) would be incomplete without mentioning the Women's Health Initiative.

Briefly, the use of Premarin and Provera as HRT caused heart attacks, strokes, breast cancer, uterine cancer and osteoporosis, not exactly what women wanted to see as side effects from a hormone replacement therapy! This happened because the hormone receptors in the hormone-derivative, Premarin (an estrogen-like substance) and Provera (a progesterone-like substance) did not fit like a key and lock. The study was intended to show how useful Premarin and Provera would have been as hormone replacement therapy; the authors hoped to show that the treatment group would live longer, have less cancer of the breast and of the uterus, have less strokes and heart attacks and would suffer less osteoporosis. But because physicians used the wrong hormone ingredients, this should not be a discouragement to continue to look for the original goals of helping women to live longer, have less postmenopausal symptoms, less cancers of the uterus and breast and no osteoporosis. The solution is simple: in Europe many women have been treated for decades with bioidentical hormones and were shown to have no postmenopausal symptoms and also no premature cardiovascular disease or cancers. You can read a 2010 review by Eileen Conaway that mentions some of today's confusion, but also points out several large European studies that did not use Premarin or Provera, but showed no increased risk of heart disease, no increased risk of cancer or osteoporosis (see references).

Diagnosis of menopause

Symptoms of hot flashes, night sweats and vaginal dryness have all been found to be strong predictors of menopause as I reviewed under references. Blood tests show that FSH and LH hormones are above the normal range when a woman is in menopause, and this is a very reliable test for menopause that your doctor can order. Usually in menopause it is the progesterone that is no longer produced by the body because the woman stopped ovulating and her ovaries do no longer produce progesterone in the missing corpus luteum that would have followed ovulation. An indirect test for progesterone depletion is a high FSH and LH blood tests as the inhibition of progesterone on the pituitary gland and the hypothalamus is missing leading to an attempt to stimulate the ovaries with FSH and LH.

Progesterone depletion is best measured directly with a saliva hormone test rather than a blood test, as progesterone in tissues accumulates to many times the value of blood tests. Only saliva tests correlate with the tissue levels of progesterone as Dr. John Lee has shown in the past (see references).

On the other hand, estrogen levels are usually well preserved in 65 to 80% of women in menopause, as the ovaries, the adrenal glands and the fatty tissue continue to produce estrogen in sufficient quantities for years to come.

Bioidentical hormone replacement (BHT)

The main principle of replacement with bioidentical hormones has been stated by Dr. John Lee and is still valid: Only replace the hormones that are missing and replace

them in the lowest possible concentration, but in the natural form, called "bioidentical". Most women in menopause will only need progesterone. This comes in many FDA approved versions, as Prometrium in 100 mg capsules taken orally, or as bioidentical progesterone cream, which is applied to the skin. You will need a prescription from a physician or naturopath. The end point of treatment is the lack of hot flashes, night sweats and vaginal dryness and the normalization of the FSH/LH blood levels. Saliva tests are expensive, but if they are taken when the other symptoms have subsided, they will also be in the normal range.

If you have problems getting these tests done and getting a prescription of the appropriate bioidentical hormone replacement, seek the advice of a naturopathic physician who is usually familiar with this type of treatment. Quite a few of the primary care physicians and gynecologists are starting to take an interest in bioidentical hormone replacement, but many of them are 20 to 30 years behind when it comes to treatment of menopause. They still recommend Premarin, which is derived from the urine of pregnant mares. These horse estrogens don't fit the human estrogen receptors, in fact they are blocking the action, and strokes, heart attacks, blood clots and osteoporosis are the consequences. No postmenopausal woman (or anybody) needs these conditions. If your doctor still recommends this prescription, maybe remind him that human females are not horses! Should you get another lecture about the "benefits" of synthetic hormones, get a second opinion from a naturopathic physician or an anti-aging physician and discuss treatment with bioidentical hormones. As a woman you have a right to be treated fairly according to the latest findings that I have described to you.

Conclusion

Bone mass density can be increased by 15% over 3 years with progesterone replacement. You can prevent heart attacks by replacing missing hormones with bioidentical ones. Apart from progesterone or testosterone levels, melatonin is often also depleted and has been found useful when replaced in attaining a better quality of sleep. Melatonin is effective in cancer prevention, so melatonin is more than a sleeping aid. The key is to not be one-sided, but to check out all your key hormones. Replace what is low with bioidentical hormones using moderation. You will have fewer symptoms; you'll live healthier, longer and will likely not develop disabilities.

The full story about testosterone

Much has been written about what happens when women get into menopause. This begs the question: do men experience a change of life? As a matter of fact, they do. It is called "andropause", the male equivalent of the menopause, and they can experience problems as a result. A study from the Massachusetts General Hospital in Boston, MA, which was published in the New England Journal of Medicine, Sept. 2013 describes in detail what happens when men get into andropause (see references).

We know from other studies that in obese men testosterone is converted into estrogen because of the enzyme aromatase that converts testosterone into estrogen resulting in erectile dysfunction and loss of sex drive. In lean men above the age of 55 there is a true testosterone reduction because the testicles produce less testosterone. This results in less sex drive, moodiness and lack of energy. But these men will do well with bioidentical testosterone replacement.

Main findings of the Massachusetts General Hospital study

Testosterone was responsible for thigh muscle development and leg press strength, for erectile function and sexual desire.

Surprisingly, estradiol, which is the main estrogen component in both sexes, plays a significant part in sexual desire in the male as well. This became particularly apparent in the post-andropause male who desired hormone replacement. When bioidentical testosterone was used to replace what's missing there was no problem with sexual desire or erectile function as a small amount of the testosterone was aromatized into estradiol. The researchers were able to measure both testosterone and estradiol levels.

Here is a surprising fact: a lack of estrogen leads to abdominal obesity. This could also be verified by hormone measurements.

In the past doctors used synthetic testosterone products like methyltestosterone, danazol, oxandrolone, testosterone propionate, testosterone cypionate or testosterone enanthate. The problem with these synthetic testosterone products is that the body cannot metabolize a portion of them into estrogen that is desirable for a normal sex drive, so the testosterone compounds alone are not doing their job as well as the bioidentical testosterone that the body can aromatize.

Obese men have too much estrogen in the system, which leads to an unbalance of the hormones in the male with a relative lack of testosterone. Overweight and obese men produce significant amounts of estrogen through aromatase located in the fatty tissue. Aromatase converts testosterone and other male type hormones, called androgens, into estrogen. Excessive levels of

estrogen cause breast growth, muscle weakness, lead to abdominal fat accumulation, heart disease and strokes. Dr. Lee described in 2003 what happens in men who enter andropause.

Testosterone to estrogen ratio

Dr. Lee indicated that in his opinion saliva hormone testing is more reliable than blood tests. One of the advantages of doing saliva hormone tests of estrogen and testosterone is that you can calculate directly the ratios of these two hormones. In hormonally normal younger males the testosterone to estrogen ratio is larger than 20 – 40. The testosterone to estrogen ratio in obese men is typically less than 20, meaning that it is too low. But lean men in andropause produce too little testosterone and their testosterone to estrogen ratio is also less than 20, because they may still have enough estrogen in their system from aromatase in the fatty tissue, but they are lacking testosterone due to a lack of its production in the testicles.

When a man in andropause is given bioidentical hormone replacement with a testosterone gel or bioidentical testosterone cream, this is absorbed into the blood and body tissues and then partially metabolized into a small amount of estrogen. This can be seen when saliva hormone tests are done; a higher level of testosterone is detected and much lower estrogen level so that the testosterone to estrogen ratio is now 20 to 40 or higher. The affected person will no longer be the "grumpy old man" that had been a source of distress to himself and the world around him.

This New England Journal of Medicine study is important, because it confirmed what anti-aging physicians had been saying for years: a small amount of estrogen is necessary for the male for bone health as estrogen receptors will regulate the bone density, it also helps for a normal sex drive. The same is true for women: a small amount of the opposite hormone - testosterone- will help a woman's sex drive, but she needs the right mix of progesterone to estrogen (a progesterone to estrogen ratio of 200:1 using saliva tests) to feel perfectly normal as a woman. You don't have to memorize any of this; I explained it to you to show you that there is more to proper bioidentical hormone replacement than meets the eye. Your experienced anti-aging physician or naturopath will know all of this and fine tune your bioidentical hormone replacement.

Health and well-being of a man depend on normal testosterone levels

It is important to realize that testosterone is not only supporting a man's sex drive and libido. Key organs like the heart, the brain and blood vessels contain testosterone receptors as well. The body of a man was designed to respond to testosterone all along. It is when testosterone production is no longer keeping up, that premature aging becomes apparent, as the target organs do no longer receive the proper signals. Randolph's website discusses this in detail (see references).

A healthy heart in a man depends on regular exercise and testosterone stimulation whether he is young, middle aged or old. The same is true for the lining of the arteries where testosterone receptors are present to help with the normal adjustment to exercise and relaxation. The brain cells have receptors for all of the sex hormones and in a man they are used to higher levels of testosterone and lower levels of progesterone and estrogen. If you take the balance away, the aging man will feel miserable and grumpy; depression will set in. Under references is a brief review how one man's life has been changed by testosterone replacement. Contrary to this news story testosterone can also be given by bioidentical cream (not by injection), which can be easily applied at home.

Bioidentical hormone replacement is not just a matter of replacing one hormone. All the hormones have to play in harmony. Lifestyle issues enter the equation as well. I have also reviewed the issue of bioidentical hormone replacement for women and men in a blog entitled "Bioidentical hormone replacement" (see references).

Conclusion

When a man reaches the age of 55 or older there comes a point where a lack of testosterone and estrogen sets in. It is wise to start doing intermittent blood or saliva hormone tests before this point is reached in order to gage when bioidentical hormone replacement treatment should be given. Along with an assessment regarding the hormone status it would be wise to also assess lifestyle issues, as often other factors play a role in premature aging. I have reviewed these factors systematically in a 2014 book entitled "A Survivor's Guide To Successful Aging", available at Amazon (see references). It is best to combine bioidentical hormone replacement with lifestyle interventions to achieve optimal preservation of a man's health. The same is true for women.

Avoid burn-out

Dr. Thierry Hertoghe, an endocrinologist from Belgium gave a lecture on "Burnout: A multiple hormone deficiency syndrome", in short: hormone changes with burnout. I have heard him speak on several congresses before. He is always very thorough and extremely knowledgeable. I decided to use this topic for this section. The lecture was presented at the 22nd Anti-Aging Congress in Las Vegas in mid December 2014.

Dr. Hertoghe said that burnout is common in teachers, soldiers, emergency room physicians and workers who have to deal with life and death situations like firefighters. In essence they burn out their hormones. In burnout several hormones are affected, with the cortisol axis being the main one. Low cortisol readings and flattening of the diurnal hormone curve can be observed in tests, but at the same time other hormone glands are affected as well. As a result endocrine glands age prematurely and symptoms of fatigue, exhaustion, gastrointestinal problems, anxiety, depression and aggressiveness develop.

When hormone levels are measured, there is a lack of cortisol, thyroid deficiency, growth hormone deficiency, testosterone/estrogen and progesterone deficiency and oxytocin deficiency. Holocaust survivors were found to have the lowest 24-hour cortisol levels. With burnout the morning output of the adrenal glands is already reduced. The health care provider must check prolactin levels, if prolactin levels are high, cortisol will be ineffective and high prolactin levels have to be addressed first. There is a questionnaire that has been originally developed for teachers called the "teacher's burnout scale" to monitor whether burnout is imminent. Soldiers who return from combative situations will also benefit from being assessed with the same test; they often suffer from burnout or from PTSD. In suspected cases hormone laboratory tests give concrete answers about hormone deficiencies.

In men growth hormone, melatonin, thyroid, testosterone, cortisol, DHEA and aldosterone have to be replaced to bring the hormone balance back to normal. Instead of

aldosterone, an adrenal gland hormone, fludrocortisone is used. In women missing hormones are replaced by bioidentical progesterone and estradiol, but small doses of testosterone are also required.

Dr. Hertoghe discussed cortisol deficiency and its replacement at some length, as this is the main stress hormone that is deficient with burnout. Different treatment protocols for cortisol replacement are used as dosing varies for different degrees of burnout. Other hormones must also be replaced as required, possibly for a prolonged period of time, if not lifelong. Supportive counseling sessions have been shown to elevate cortisol levels and several studies were discussed. A counselor or psychiatrist will help to tone down increased brain activity and help regain the internal balance. Balanced hormones are necessary on a cellular level to regulate the metabolism of every cell in the body.

Hormone balance and symptoms of various deficiencies

Cortisol is placed on one side of the scales and is balanced by androgens (DHEA), estrogens in women and testosterone in men, growth hormone and melatonin on the other side of the scales. When fainting is part of the burnout, it is because of extremely low aldosterone from the adrenal glands. The best treatment for this is fludrocortisone, which will bring the blood pressure up and remove the hazardous symptom of fainting. Symptoms of "slow thinking, slow moving" and tiredness are often from hypothyroidism. The best treatment for this is T3/T4 (Armour thyroid) treatment. Many physicians still use either T3 or T4, which is not physiological. The body manufactures a mix of T3 and T4,

so the bioidentical replacement should be a T3/T4 product. Symptoms of "poor resistance to noise" are due to DHEA deficiency. In addition DHEA deficiency often is associated with moderately poor resistance to stress and joint aches called arthralgias.

When permanent fatigue is present, it is time to measure sex hormone levels. If deficiencies are found in a woman, bioidentical estrogen known as Bi-Est is given transdermally from day 5 to 25 of the cycle, and progesterone transdermally from day 15 to 25 of her cycle. Depending on how severe the hormone deficiency is, hormone replacement doses in women range from 2.5 to 5.0 mg for bioidentical estrogen and from 100 mg to 150-200mg for bioidentical progesterone per day.

Sports fatigue

In the age of exaggerated sports activities a new entity of burnout, the sports fatigue has emerged. A low free testosterone/cortisol ratio is a reliable marker for overtraining. When this ratio shows a decrease of 30% or more, it shows that there is a temporarily incomplete recovery from intensive training. In the lab often an increase in the sex hormone-binding globulin (SHBG) can be measured, which leads to a lack of free testosterone. In a study of Chinese over-trained soldiers there was a complete recovery from this sports fatigue with multi-vitamins and a liposomal testosterone gel.

Sleep abnormalities

Restless, non-restorative sleep can be a symptom of melatonin deficiency and happens more often in people above the age of 50. There is a natural hormone decline with age in the older generation. Treatment consists of

replacement, which is easily achieved either with sublingual tablets (mild: 0.05mg, moderate: 0.15 to 0.5 mg, severe: 0.5 to 1mg) or oral tablets. Oral melatonin doses are more problematical, as there are average absorbers and poor absorbers. For mild, moderate to severe symptoms of insomnia the sublingual melatonin dosages for average absorbers are 0.2mg, 1 mg and 2 mg and for poor absorbers 0.3mg, 1.5mg and 10mg. One should use the lowest effective dose of melatonin as it opposes cortisol and when melatonin is overused, adrenal gland weakness with lower cortisol production could develop.

Exhaustion

An overpowering feeling of exhaustion can be due to growth hormone (GH) deficiency. This is diagnosed by testing insulin-like growth factor-1 (IGF-1) level in the blood. When this is low, daily subcutaneous injection of low-dose human growth hormone is given. Depending on how severe growth hormone deficiency is, different GH doses are administered. The patient self-injects with an insulin injector. Mild GH deficiency requires 0.05 mg (1 click) per day, moderate deficiency 0.1 mg (2 clicks) per day and severe deficiency 0.15 mg (3 clicks) per day. In order to give the body a rest, many physicians recommend a break of two weeks, so the treatment is two weeks on, two weeks off preventing overdosing with growth hormone. Howwever, if the IGF-1 level dose not come up, daily injections may have to be given. Lately a new test, a 24-hour urine test for growth hormone metabolites has been introduced that is more accurate than IGF-1. Both growth hormone and growth hormone testing are very expensive at this time.

Adrenaline deficiency

Dr. Hertoghe pointed out with the help of a publication where runners had developed overtraining syndrome that adrenaline deficiency can be part of burnout. A laboratory test on these runners showed that overnight catecholamine, which is the metabolized adrenaline excretion, was only 50% of healthy runners. Often this is associated with thyroid deficiencies in males and females, or with estrogen deficiency in women. The approach is to rectify the thyroid and sex hormone deficiencies by estradiol and progesterone replacement in women.

Treatment of burnout

Dr. Hertoghe suggested a 5-step treatment protocol.

1.Improve your diet

This involves the removal of sugar and starch as both lower the levels of essential hormones. Dr. Hertoghe emphasized that sweets, chocolate drinks, soft drinks, milk, bread, pasta, commercial mueslis and high temperature cooked meats need to disappear from the diet plan.

The consumption of animal protein is desirable, but the food should be cooked at low temperatures. Fresh vegetable and fruit consumption should be increased. I like to add that these foods are best consumed as organic foods. These foods will increase your natural hormones and produce energy in your cells.

2. Improve your sleep

This requires a dark bedroom at night and day light exposure in the morning. Avoid TV's, electrical alarm

clocks, i-phones and computers at the bedside. For sensitive individuals EMF can be sleep- disturbing. If your environment is noisy, you may require earplugs to shut out the noise. In case of hormone deficiency, it may be necessary to replace missing melatonin, growth hormone, or the other hormones mentioned above. Progesterone is important in women and oxytocin can also play a role.

3. Treat adrenal deficiency, if present

The missing hormones here to be replaced are cortisol, DHEA and often aldosterone, (being replaced with fludrocortisone).

4. Treat other associated hormone deficiencies

The other hormones, which are often overlooked, are growth hormone, thyroid hormones, estradiol/progesterone in women and testosterone in men.

5. Treat nutritional deficiencies

The most common missing minerals and vitamins are iron, magnesium, folic acid, vitamin B12, vitamin E and others. Replacement of these along with the missing hormones is essential for normal cell function.

Conclusion

In an attempt to add to our physical fitness we may overlook our limits and run into a burnout situation without noticing it. Your medical care provider should think about multiple hormone and nutritional deficiencies that can be treated, although treatment can be multifaceted. If in doubt, ask for a referral to an anti-aging physician or naturopath.

Grumpiness

Researchers in a study from Finland found that grumpiness in older age seems to lead to dementia at a faster rate. I like to emphasize that there may be an underlying problem of hormone deficiency as well.

Other studies have shown that in males low testosterone levels are associated with grumpiness, and dementia is setting in sooner in those males who are deficient for testosterone. For older grumpy females it is the lack of progesterone that has been found to be deficient and when you replace it, memory comes back, symptoms of menopause reverse themselves and the grumpiness is gone. Testosterone replacement may be required in as many as 1 in 4 men in the their 40's as is summarized in an article from Great Britain.

How can we tell whether there is a change in an older man? This publication from the Yucatan Times points to quite a few symptoms that can be seen by loved ones surrounding around this man: an increase in abdominal girth, shrinking muscles, lack of energy, irritability (see references). The key is to convince the patient to consult a doctor and ask the doctor to order a bioavailable testosterone blood test.

According to medical research 84% of men and 62% of women in the age group of 57 to 64 have been sexually active in the previous 12 months. Take an older age group of 65 to 74 and still 67% of men and 40% of women are sexually active. Fast-forward to age 75 to 85 and the rate has dropped to 39% of men and 17% of women. A person's sexual activity is like a barometer that indicates how well the hormones are balanced. These figures show that bioidentical hormone replacement has not been well accepted. Women have a reason to be cautious as Big

Pharma as was shown in the Women's Health Initiative misled them.

Women's Health Initiative

The National Institutes of Health had funded a large study, the Women's Health Initiative, to clarify what was going on with regard to side effects and effects of HRT. HRT stands for hormone replacement therapy.

Unfortunately, synthetic non-bioidentical hormone products were used in these studies, namely Premarin and Provera, instead of bioidentical estrogen and progesterone. The results of the Women's Health Initiative were devastating. In 2002 doctors were warned by the National Institute of Health that Premarin and Provera used for HRT would cause increased heart attack rates and breasts cancer, which led to premature deaths. Overall the placebo group did better than the experimental group and this is why the trial was prematurely stopped. As a result of the wide publicity regarding the negative results of the Women's Health Initiative postmenopausal women either do not see their physician for hormone replacement or are advised by conventional doctors that only small amounts of Premarin could be used for not more than 5 years for fear of causing breast cancer. Medico-legal considerations are at play and the whole issue of HRT after menopause has been politicized.

Problems now for HRT

It is like a negative shadow that has been cast forward with regard to hormone replacement because of the Women's Health Initiative. People are still confused and don't understand that the synthetic hormone-like drugs from Big Pharma are like an ill-fitting key for the hormone receptors in the body, whereas bioidentical hormones are the perfect fit.

Otherwise there would not be a 45% drop-off from 62% to 17% in sexual activities in women from the age of 60 to 80. Men have it somewhat easier: their drop rate between age 60 and 80 is also 45% from 84% to 39%, but as they entered into andropause 10 to 15 years later than women did with menopause, their sexual activity is still double that of women at the age of 80.

However, if people could overcome their unrealistic fear of bioidentical hormones, hormones that fit the body's hormone receptors, a lot more people would be encouraged to use bioidentical hormone replacements. This would normalize the sex drive for both men and women and would prevent a lot of difficulties in personal intimate relationships.

What if the grumpy old man is willing to see his doctor?

The doctor should look at all of the hormones including a fasting insulin level as hyperinsulinism often complicates hormone replacement. Thyroid hormones, which often are also lowered at an older age, should be tested as well; so the doctor would order a T3, T4 and TSH level. A saliva hormone test can show a panel of 5 hormones: cortisol, DHEAS, testosterone, progesterone and estradiol. As hormones are in a balance with each other this allows computing the testosterone to estrogen ratio, which ought to be 20 or higher. But hormones alone are not the answer. Administration of hormones needs to be combined with proper nutrition. As already mentioned, cut out sugar, starchy foods, preferably switch to organic foods to escape the xenoestrogens that foul up your hormone balance; also engage in regular exercise and use vitamins and supplements. I have summarized all of this in my 2014 book “A survivor’s Guide to Successful Aging” (see references).

When the hormone tests come back, the doctor will likely give you a prescription for the missing hormones, hopefully as bioidentical hormones! These are usually applied as a vanishing cream on the forearms or on the chest wall above the breasts.

It can take 2 to 3 months before the full effect of bioidentical hormone replacement is seen. But most men will be astounded how well they can feel. The patient will notice that he does not tire with exercising. His muscle mass builds up, and his posture will improve. His stamina will come back. He will find that the previously foggy thinking is gone, and his thought processes have become clear again. And yes, his sex live comes back. So now he has to talk to his sex partner about her bioidentical hormone replacement so they both can enjoy the benefits!

Hidden benefits of bioidentical hormone replacement

The bones become stronger, the heart becomes stronger and better, the brain thinks clearer, because the key organs like the brain, the heart and the bones have the appropriate hormone receptors in both sexes. No, this is no exaggeration. Heart function can be measured by an exercise tolerance test. Bone density can be measured; this has been done and it showed a 2% to 4% increase per year! Brain function is indirectly visible to the people around the person: apart from new vitality, improvements in mood and more energy, the grumpiness is gone and the person is perceived as being his normal self once again.

Conclusion

The observation of an "old, grumpy man" when he entered the male menopause is accurate, but this should not distract from the fact that he has a responsibility to look after himself. It is important to recognize that it is not only women who enter the menopause. Men are not exempt from aging, but for them the same difficulties appear 10 to 15 years later. Both sexes enter a state of hormone unbalance that is treatable. The answer is to replace the hormone deficiency with the missing bioidentical hormones.

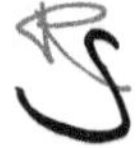

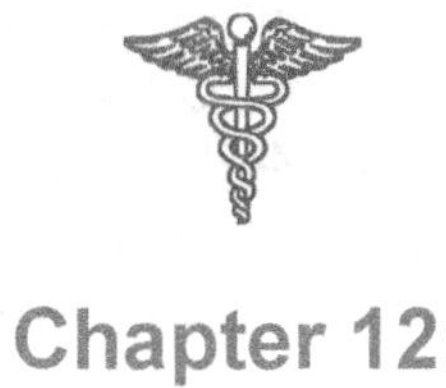

Chapter 12:

General Thoughts on Anti-Aging

Anti-aging has become a hot topic in the past few years. It is a branch of medicine that wants to help stabilize our metabolism so that aging is slowed down and the risk for diseases and disabilities is minimized.

We will start reviewing the mitochondria, a small sub particle within the cells that provides our energy. We briefly reviewed mitochondria in chapter 4. It is in the mitochondria where the energy metabolism takes place. Following this we will start to review "Stem cells/lifestyle/ telomeres/hormones and stress". After this overview we will learn more details about telomeres; it is known that longer telomeres make us live longer. I will review what supplements you can take to elongate your telomeres and what you should avoid. This leads us to lifestyle and how that affects telomeres. For instance, smoking is one of the things that shorten telomeres and life. It is not only deaths from lung cancer/other cancers, heart attacks and emphysema that kills people who smoke, it is the shortening of telomeres in all body cells leading to organ failures of the key organs. Lifestyle has an enormous impact on our telomeres: exercise and a Mediterranean diet with olive oil will lengthen our telomeres and help us live longer.

One section will deal with focusing on health rather than disease. We then move on to review how we can prevent 40% of premature deaths.

Nothing good comes from sitting back and letting nature take its course. We need to put a little effort into creating longevity; what we do now for ourselves will make a significant difference for us later in life. When you are a senior, you can hopefully reap the benefits of good health by having exercised, eaten the right foods and done everything right in the previous decades. You should continue to have energy, do things you enjoy, move about and carry on with an exercise program, go dancing or enjoy other physical activities. I expect you to stay active and stay disease free.

Mitochondrial DNA

New research on mitochondria has shown that "frail mitochondrial DNA equals frail people". More specifically, researchers from the McKusick-Nathans Institute of Genetic Medicine of the Johns Hopkins University School of Medicine in Baltimore, MD found that mitochondrial DNA content varies according to age with less mitochondrial DNA in older age. Women have an advantage over men in that they have multiple mitochondrial DNA copies , more so than men. Mitochondrial DNA has an inverse relationship to frailty and a direct relationship to life expectancy.

Mitochondria are the powerhouses within each cell, and there are between 10 and several thousand mitochondria per cell, depending on what the power needs of a cell type are. Brain and heart cells are two examples where there are thousands of mitochondria per cell.

Each mitochondrion has its own mitochondrial DNA contained in 2 to 10 small circular chromosomes that regulate the 37 genes necessary for normal mitochondrial function.

In order to track mitochondrial DNA and its relationship to frailty and old age, the Johns Hopkins University researchers accessed data from two large clinical trials. One study was the Cardiovascular Health Study (CHS), which took place between 1989 and 2006. The other one was the Atherosclerosis Risk in Communities (ARIC) study spanning from 1987 to 2013. Blood tests were available on participants from both studies that allowed determinations of mitochondrial DNA.

In multi ethnic groups it was apparent that mitochondrial DNA content was dictated by the age of a person.

Frailty was defined as a person who had aging symptoms including weakness, a lack of energy compared to the past, activity levels that were much lower than before and loss of weight. When persons with frailty as defined by these criteria were identified in the two studies, they were found to have 9% less mitochondrial DNA than nonfrail study participants.

Another subgroup were white participants; when their bottom mitochondrial DNA content was compared to the top mitochondrial DNA content, the researchers found that frailty was 31% more common in the bottom DNA content group. This means that white people are more prone to frailty and they should take steps early on to prevent this.

Mortality data were also examined, and it turned out that those study participants who had the highest level of mitochondrial DNA lived 2.1 years longer on average than those with the lowest level of mitochondrial DNA. It is the amount of mitochondrial DNA that matters.

The study also found that women in the two clinical trials had 21% more DNA in their mitochondria on average than men, which explains that as a group women generally outlive males.

Prevention of DNA loss from mitochondria

The study did not suggest any preventative steps against mitochondrial DNA loss. But there is ample evidence in the literature that this can be achieved through supplements that can both help multiply mitochondria as well as stimulate the metabolism of mitochondria. Lifestyle changes are also effective.

I am not supporting any specific brands of supplements, but find the common sense explanations of Dr. Whitaker very useful, as they explain what the supplements do. You find a link to Dr. Whitaker's site under references.

You may find the scientific data too tedious to delve into, but let this list be of help to you to preserve your health and vitality:

1. Mitochondrial aging is slowed down by ubiquinol (=Co-Q-10, I take 400 mg per day). Co-Q-10 repairs DNA damage to your mitochondria.

2. Another supplement, 20 mg of PQQ (=Pyrroloquinoline quinone) per day stimulates your healthy mitochondria to multiply. Between the two supplements you will have more energy as optimal mitochondrial function is ensured. Exercise more and regularly as this will also stimulate your mitochondria to multiply similar to the effects of PQQ.

3. There are simple lifestyle changes you can make: eat less calories as this will stimulate SIRT1 genes, which in turn stimulates your cell metabolism including the mitochondria.

4. Resveratrol, the supplement from red grape skin can also stimulate your mitochondria metabolism. I take

500mg of trans-Resveratrol once daily. This is a powerful antioxidant that protects mitochondria from free radical damage.

5. Alpha-lipoic acid (often abbreviated as ALA) is an anti-oxidant that counters the slow-down of mitochondrial metabolism. I recommend 300mg per day.

6. L-arginine is an amino acid that is a precursor of nitric oxide (NO). In older age the enzyme for conversion to nitric oxide may be missing. Red beet is known to stimulate nitric oxide production from the lining of the arteries.

7. Hawthorn is an herb that has been found useful for prevention of heart disease and treatment of mild heart failure (in Germany known as "Crataegutt"). It has been found to be endothelium protective and may stimulate mitochondria. 150 to 500 mg once daily is a preventative dose.

Caution is needed to discern between salesmanship and science regarding mitochondrial support, but this overview should start you off in the right direction. You can get all of these supplements in any health food store.

Telomere length a telltale sign of aging

1. Dr. Sandy Chang gave a talk at the 22nd Annual World Congress on Anti-Aging Medicine in Las Vegas Dec. 10-14, 2014 entitled "Telomere measurement as a diagnostic Test in cardiovascular and Age-related disease", but a shorter title would be "telomere length a telltale sign of aging" (my choosing).

Dr. Chang pointed out that it is now well established that telomere length is directly related to health. The

shorter the telomeres are the higher the probability to get the following: early menopause, infertility, diabetes, wrinkles, arthritis, osteoporosis, cardiovascular disease, Alzheimer's, Parkinson's, dementia, cancer, stress and a lack of stem cells. In a BMJ study from 2014 it was shown on a large population basis that shorter white blood cell telomeres lead to a higher risk of coronary heart disease causing heart attacks. Decreased telomere length is also associated with the development of breast cancer, cancer of the ovaries and uterus, cancer of the prostate and skin cancer.

Because of these connections it makes sense to determine a person's telomere length. If the telomeres are short, do check-ups more often to detect any cancer early, when it can still be successfully treated.

Telomere length measurements are now done in many infertility clinics, as short telomeres both in the male and female are associated with infertility.

The newest finding and perhaps the most important is that a healthy lifestyle, vitamins and supplements can elongate telomeres while a poor lifestyle leads to shortening of telomeres.

Here are the factors that lead to shortening of telomeres:

- **Chronic stress**
- **Poor diet and nutritional habits**
- **Chronic inflammatory diseases**
- **Metabolic disorders**
- **Lack of consistent exercise/sedentary lifestyle**
- **Obesity, high BMI and body fat**
- **Smoking**
- **Over consumption of alcohol**
- **Lack of sleep / insomnia**

When short telomeres are detected, it is important for the physician recommend lifestyle changes to the patient. This will protect telomeres from decreasing their length even further. This has the potential of preventing dementia and Alzheimer's when it comes to brain health. It can prevent osteoporosis and metabolic diseases like diabetes and metabolic syndrome. Telomerase is the buzzword today, which is an enzyme that all of our cells have. The purpose why we have telomerase in our cells seems to be helping us build up and repair telomeres. Any substance that preserves telomerase or prevents the breakdown of telomerase will prevent shortening of telomeres and will also prevent the above-mentioned diseases.

These supplements lead to lengthening of telomeres:

- Vitamin C and E
- Omega-3 and polyphenols
- Vitamin A and vitamin D3
- All of these help controlling oxidative stress, reduce DNA damage, reduce inflammation and build up telomere length.
- A good diet and nutrition like a Mediterranean type diet will prevent telomere shortening and even leads to telomere lengthening.
- T-65, an extract from astragalus has been shown in vitro to lengthen telomeres, but there is no publication yet about in vivo effects in humans.
- Resveratrol is useful to prevent shortening of telomeres as well.
- Exercise is a simple means to prevent telomere shortening.

2. Another talk on telomeres was given by Dr. Harvey Bartnof at the 22nd Annual World Congress on Anti-Aging

Medicine in Las Vegas Dec. 10-14, 2014 with the title "Telomere Shortening and Modulation: Case Studies From The Clinic".

This talk was a comprehensive review of what is known about telomeres, about the fact that many diseases are due to telomere shortening, about animal experiments, ways of how to lengthen telomeres and finally some data on human studies with regard to telomere lengthening.

In the following I will briefly review all of these areas that were discussed. Some of this material overlaps with Dr. Chang's lecture and I have left out duplications as much as possible.

What produces telomere shortening? Dr. Bartnof showed 4 slides that listed all of the conditions and diseases that are associated with telomere shortening.

Telomere shortening doubles the risk of dying from a heart attack when compared to people with normal telomeres.

a) Known genetic conditions in humans associated with telomere shortening

There are three known genetic conditions due to telomere shortening: A premature aging syndrome, called *dyskeratosis congenitalis*; patients with this condition die prematurely from cancer, or from bone marrow failure.

People with *Werner syndrome* who have a genetic telomere loss have a mean life expectancy of only 54 years.

***Idiopathic pulmonary fibrosis* is another genetic condition with shortened telomeres due to mutations. Patients who develop this condition usually die from respiratory failure 3 to 5 years following the development of pulmonary fibrosis.**

b) Telomere shortening associated with these health conditions

Professor Elizabeth Blackburn, PhD who is one of the three researchers who won the Nobel Prize in Physiology and Medicine for their work on telomeres in 2009 stated the following: "Telomere shortness is associated with just about all the major diseases of aging… from cardiovascular disease, death from cardiovascular disease, risks of cardiovascular disease, diabetes, diabetes risks such as insulin resistance, vascular dementia, to osteoarthritis."

An enormous amount of clinical investigations have been done since in cohort groups like people with diabetes, high blood pressure, obesity and cancer.

There is also natural shortening of telomeres due to the aging process. When we compare telomere length of body cells of a 20-year old and call this 100%, the telomeres of a 100-year old person are on average only 40%. A study from the Karolinska Institute found in a group of matching twins where one twin had shortened telomeres, this twin had a 2.8 times greater risk of death than the twin with normal telomere length.

However, as already mentioned, a number of other factors can lead to shorter telomeres like chronic stress in workers who look after Alzheimer patients, being of the Caucasian race (compared to African-American), having had less education, chronic unemployment, depression, pessimism, single people versus married people, phobic anxiety in women and hostility in men, poor sleep and too little sleep, migraine headaches in women, low physical activity, smoking cigarettes and alcohol consumption. The list does not stop here. Other conditions are associated with telomere shortening like heroin abuse, exposure to smog, polycyclic aromatic hydrocarbons and lead,

cardiovascular disease, diabetes, cancers, osteoporosis, osteoarthritis, rheumatoid arthritis, cirrhosis of the liver, inflammatory bowel disease, chronic obstructive lung disease (emphysema), Alzheimer's disease, Parkinson's disease, chronic kidney disease and disability in the elderly.

c) Effects of medications on telomere length

Antidepressants used against depression have a telomere lengthening effect, but NSAID's, aspirin and interferon-alpha shorten telomeres. Other telomere shortening effects come from cancer chemotherapy.

d) Telomerase activation elongates telomeres

Successful experiments in various mouse strains showed that special strains that were telomerase deficient, could be reconstituted to normal by reinserting telomerase: atrophied organs regrew back to normal size and function. In humans it was shown that increased physical activity elongated telomeres, so did vitamin C, E and vitamin D3 supplementation, resveratrol, a Mediterranean diet, marine omega-3 fatty acid supplementation, higher fiber intake, bioidentical estrogen in women and testosterone in men, relaxation techniques like yoga and meditation. The Astragalus-derived telomerase activator TA-65 has been shown in animal experiments to elongate telomeres. The human data about TA-65 is still spotty or not available. It is also very expensive and may not even be necessary, given the fact that so many other agents are known to lengthen telomeres.

e) Human data on telomere lengthening

Much can be achieved by changing one's lifestyle. It has been mentioned before: cut out toxins like cigarette

smoking and alcohol abuse. Get involved in a regular exercise program, which has been shown to increase HDL cholesterol and to elongate telomeres. Adopt a Mediterranean type diet including olive oil; take vitamin E, D, C and supplements with resveratrol and marine omega-3 fatty acids, all of which elongate telomeres. Get enough sleep (7 to 8 hours per night) and do yoga and meditation. Avoid distress and tone down your stress level to eustress (normal stress level associated with everyday living). An older person should use bioidentical hormones to replace missing hormones. All of this taken together will create a milieu in your body where telomeres get elongated, and you live longer without disease. Several clinical conditions were mentioned where baseline telomere length was assessed initially and the telomeres were found to be too short. Simple lifestyle changes were then initiated, which were able to improve telomere length and treat these diseases successfully. In addition TA-65 (also termed T-65) was given in some of these cases, but in a subsequent discussion Dr. Bartnof admitted that he could not comment on how effective TA-65 by itself was as it was only one component of many other effective telomerase stimulators given. Till further research is published regarding this substance, it may be too costly without spectacular benefits on its own.

Conclusion

I gave a summary of the talks by Dr. Chang and Dr. Bartnof regarding telomeres, but these were not the only talks about telomeres, although quite representative for the others. Both speakers pointed out how powerful lifestyle is for our body functions as this is what lengthens our telomeres and allows us to live longer, disease-free lives. Stem cells also have telomeres, but they are on average longer than the rest of the body cells, called somatic cells. An improved lifestyle will keep our stem cells in good shape, so they are there when needed to replace aging somatic cells.

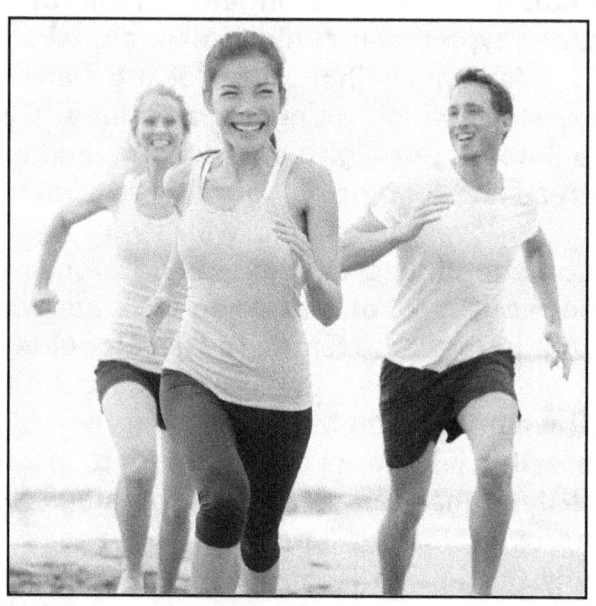

The new logic of a healthy lifestyle

A healthy lifestyle causes healthy telomeres of somatic cells and of stem cells; this causes health until a ripe old age.

More on lifestyle

Dr. David Katz delivered a keynote address at the 22nd Annual World Congress on Anti-Aging Medicine in Las Vegas Dec. 10-14, 2014 entitled "Integrative Medicine: A Bridge Over Healthcare's Troubled Waters".

He started the 1-hour talk with showing a slide of six blind men and the elephant. He concluded that each of the blind men saw only one aspect of the elephant, but no one saw the true elephant. With healthcare it is a bit like that.

Back in 1993 McGinnis list was published that showed the ten factors that were responsible for chronic disease, but the first three things on the McGinnis list were the most important ones: tobacco use, diet and lack of exercise.

Already several years back, various researchers found damaging factors and reported about them, such as smoking. Dr. Katz said: “Although there is no magic pill for reducing disease, lifestyle is exactly ‘the magic pill’ that reduces mortality by 80%.”

Nothing has changed in 2014. The authors still come to the same conclusion when examining what would be able to prevent heart attacks. All of them stated that LIFESTYLE is what matters.

We live in the “epigenetic age: dinner is destiny!” With this Dr. Katz meant to say that our genes get switched on and off depending on what we put into our mouths. This determines whether we live shorter or longer lives, stay healthy or have to struggle with illnesses and disability.

He went on to say: “Feet (exercise), forks (diet), fingers (cigarettes) are what matters.” Oncogenes can get turned off in prostate cancer with the help of exercise, the right food intake and quitting smoking.

Dr. Katz mentioned the book by Michael Moss “Salt, sugar, fat”, which made it to the cover story of Time Magazine in 2013. In it is described how the food industry employs PhD’s to include agents in processed foods to ensure that consumers get addicted to their food products. Food addiction leads to obesity; the CDC statistics show that it is effective. We have put up with this for far too long. There are differences of obesity rates between countries: in a link from the CDC under references shows a comparison between Canadian and US obesity statistics.

Dr. Katz asked the audience to raise their hands, if they had a person close to them die of cancer, a heart attack or a stroke. Almost all of the more than 500 participants in the hall raised their hands.

So what is the ONE thing that can fix everything? He answered this rhetoric question by saying that there is no "one thing that fixes everything". But we can start at a young age by educating our children. Dr. Katz has started a program for school kids called "ABC for fitness for kids" to prevent obesity. The program teaches children healthful food choices. Many of these can also be found on YouTube. Dr. Katz said: "Kids speak YouTube". Dr. Katz commented further that a website, NuVal uses a nutritional value rating system to monitor food quality and manufacturers have improved the content of their products because the composition of their products were displayed on that website. We need to be vigilant and read labels.

But we can only change one thing at a time, like we walk one step at a time on a spiral staircase to get to the next floor. We ask ourselves about our lifestyle: what is the first thing to fix? We may decide that we have to exercise instead of parking ourselves on the couch. Then we fix the second point: adopt a Mediterranean diet. The third step would be taking specific vitamins and supplements. In other words, we approach one thing at a time or things will become overwhelming. Integrative medicine, the fusion of conventional and non-conventional medicine, can help to solve problems one step at a time. Despite a bias in the North American medical literature saying that CoQ10 was "useless", the European Heart Journal reported in 2013 that CoQ10 decreases all-cause-mortality in patients with heart disease. A more recent article from Dec. 2014 regarding a two-year trial with congestive heart failure patients taking only 100 mg of CoQ-10 three times daily found that all-cause-mortality was reduced significantly.

There is a new wave going around the United States: it is the idea to copy the lifestyle of the blue zones around the world. Blue zones are areas in the world where the life expectancy is 100 years or more. There is a video about blue zones that is worth watching.

It explains how Blue Zones are being established all around America. Dr. Katz explained that *lifestyle is the medicine* and the *environment is the spoon*. In Blue Zones it is the environment that influences people in a positive fashion to live in wellness and health. Often the examples are conveyed non-verbally. Organic vegetables in stores are cheaper in Blue Zones, so it is easier to eat more of them; people socialize more with each other, they exercise more and dance. This is what people do who live longer than 100 years. In other words, you change the culture, you change your lifestyle, you exercise more, you stop smoking, you eat healthy and you live longer.

Dr. Katz ended his lecture with the image of you walking along and coming to a fork. To go further you must now decide to go on the pathway to your right or on the pathway to the left. You turn on the right pathway by deciding to adopt the principles of the Blue Zones; you make the decision to want to turn older than 100 years and keep your vitality until it is time for you to pass on. In the meantime you enjoy every day, you are not disabled, and your mind and body stay healthy. The other pathway was the one that the majority of the industrialized Western nations have taken in the last few decades. Which path will it be that you decide to take?

Conclusion

At the conference Dr. Katz and a number of other speakers pointed out how powerful a healthy lifestyle is for our body functions. Other speakers stressed the importance of telomeres, the caps of the chromosomes, which comprise the end of the double stranded DNA. With every cell division our telomeres shorten. Stem cells also have telomeres, but they are on average longer than the somatic dells. Both, the stem cells and the somatic cells have the enzyme telomerase, which can elongate telomeres given the proper lifestyle. The stem cells' job is to replace the aging somatic cells for as long as possible.

Remember: a healthy lifestyle causes healthy telomeres of somatic cells and of stem cells; this causes health until a ripe old age. I will discuss this further below.

Focus on health

Not too long ago I came across a blog that summarized the "18 Biggest Problems with Modern Medicine". Although this is a useful list, it occurred to me that these problems could be compressed into about 9 underlying themes. Below I am describing the same type of problems regarding modern medicine in a somewhat abbreviated fashion.

1. The patient is seen as a complicated machine with parts that could break down. When there is a breakdown of the machinery, symptoms develop, which are quickly fixed with a patented medicine, but without really addressing the underlying problem.

This type of approach soothes pain, but changes nothing for a chronic illness like MS. Nobody has all the answers to this complicated illness, but we know that it is an autoimmune disease. So it makes sense to avoid foods that could make the patient worse. This is exactly what Dr. Terry Wahls is describing in her YouTube video.

Also, vitamins and supplements for multiple sclerosis that support the immune system would be useful. Vitamin D3 in high doses with monitoring of blood levels by doing 25-hydroxy vitamin D blood tests from time to time would also be useful.

2. A holistic approach to building up health rather than fixing a clinical problem, which belongs to a disease, is not part of modern medicine.

In the past a stomach acid problem was treated with H-2 receptor antagonists like cimetidine or ranitidine. The newer proton pump inhibitors, like omeprazole were added and were supposed to be better in suppressing the acid formation. But they did nothing to cure the ulcer or gastritis problem. The problem often was that chronic stress allowed a bacterium, H. pylori to multiply in the stomach wall causing stomach acid and a burning sensation. This did respond to the antacid medications for a period of time, but it came back when the medication was stopped. A simple over the counter licorice compound, called DGL or mastic gum from the health food store can cure the helicobacter infection and cure your peptic ulcer disease without the need for the expensive patented H-2 receptor antagonists or proton pump inhibitors. These simple remedies are available in health food stores. They are called "Licorice compound or DGL" and "Mastic gum".

3. Everybody with the same disease is treated with the same medical treatment schedule, often agreed on by consensus expert panels. The body's self-healing capacity or the placebo effect, which is an expression of the same natural healing response, is ignored.

Here is a study that was done on patients with irritable bowel syndrome (IBS) on placebo pills (see references). Placebo pills were 24% more effective than the control group who took no pills in controlling symptoms of IBS. Why not utilize the power of belief (placebo pills) in conventional medicine?

4. The disease is treated, not the patient; numbers from lab tests count, not clinical signs of the physical examination. What used to be called the "art of medicine" has been abandoned.

The art of medicine is important to establish a rapport with the patient, but also to pick up on silent features during the examination that may otherwise be overlooked.

5. Diet, lifestyle, hormone changes, which are due to chronic stress and older age, are all ignored. If there are the hormone changes of menopause or andropause, only synthetic hormones are given and only for a limited time not exceeding 5 years. Bioidentical hormone replacement invokes butterfly feelings in the physician's stomach and must therefore be rejected. It's almost a knee-jerk response. The reason for that is the fear that bioidentical hormones would have the same devastating side effects as the synthetic hormones. However, this is a fallacy, as a young person with fully functioning natural hormones will not come down with nefarious side effects of strokes, heart attacks or cancer.

You can read interesting facts about bioidentical hormones on a website by Dr. Lee (see references).

6. It is a sad fact that our bodies may have been exposed to toxins like heavy metals, xenoestrogens etc. from the environment that are taken up and stored in the body like a sponge. It stands to reason to use detoxification from time to time. But this approach is foreign thinking to modern medicine except for a small group of dedicated physicians and naturopaths who offer various forms of chelation therapy.

The TART trial has shown that there was an 18% reduction of heart attack rates in the group that received 40 chelation therapy treatments. Chelation therapy can easily be combined with traditional treatment methods, but conventional medicine mostly ignores this option.

7. Similarly the idea that supplements and vitamins would be essential to support the body in the fight against free radicals that form inside the body every day is not something every doctor will feel comfortable in recommending.

In my 2014 book I have cited evidence from a clinical trial that multivitamins elongate telomeres by 5.1% and add 9.8 years of productive life in those who take multivitamins over a long period of time versus those who do not.

8. In the health care industry we are still working in a hierarchical system where the doctor is on top and the patient is on a lower level and dependent. In the future medical system the doctor and the patient are equal partners who try to solve a health problem as a team.

The doctor may have more experience in diagnosing, prescribing and monitoring health problems, but the patient is the one who owns the problem and is encouraged to comply with the prescribed treatment and to report back to the doctor, if there are new symptoms that may lead the doctor to new insights resulting in improving the treatment plan.

9. Big Pharma influences doctors to prescribe their patented medicines. New drugs and old drugs are sold like the latest invention against the dreaded disease XYZ - you can fill in whatever the diagnosis is! But none of these drugs is effective against a hormone unbalance, stress, a lack of sleep, lack of exercise or malnutrition. The patient's co-operation is needed to work on these issues.

I have explained that the metabolic syndrome, which is responsible for much of our modern diseases (diabetes, heart attacks, arthritis, strokes, cancers, Alzheimer's disease) can be overcome by a combination of steps: paying attention to our food intake, cutting out sugar and high glycemic starchy foods and excessive , unhealthy fats as explained in my 2014 book. Regular exercise will help you to build up and maintain muscle mass and at the same time melt in excessive fat. Yoga, self-hypnosis, meditation and prayer can remedy stress. Bioidentical hormones can replace any hormone deficiencies. Detoxification, vitamins and supplements complete this program, which allows you to successfully age without disabilities. All these steps taken together allow your body to recover and find a new balance where drugs are rarely needed.

Conclusion

The reason Medicare is so expensive is that life style issues are not often addressed. If only symptoms are treated and the underlying causes of an illness are not removed the illness will not be cured. Look at heart attacks as an example: If you want to go down the road from angina to heart attack to bypass surgery or stents, you will soon run out of options. The next level of curative medicine approach is a heart transplant after heart attack number 4 or 5. Comprehensive medicine would approach this differently by paying attention to what you eat and motivate you to cut out starchy foods, wheat, and sugar. This would address obesity, which is a problem in many Western countries. You would engage in regular physical exercise, which alone has been shown to cut heart attack rates by 50%! Stress would be overcome in yoga classes or self-hypnosis sessions. Bioidentical hormones would replace your missing hormones based on saliva hormone tests or blood test samples. The heart muscle that has a lot of testosterone receptors would respond to this. As mentioned above, a series of chelation treatments to remove heavy metals could also be offered in this combined, comprehensive heart attack prevention program with a reduction of another 18% of heart attacks. This all is available now and combined will cut down 90% of heart attacks, but regrettably few people make use of it.

Prevent 40% of premature deaths

A new report from the CDC (Center of Disease Control) in the US has revealed that up to 40% of premature deaths could be prevented by simple lifestyle changes. As the link under references shows every year about 900,000 premature deaths occur in the US, which are due to 5 major diseases that in the opinion of the CDC can be prevented by 20 to 40%. Here are the diseases that kill:

- Cancer
- Heart disease
- COPD/emphysema
- Stroke
- Accidents/injuries

These conditions were responsible for 63% of all deaths in the US in 2010. Let's discuss each of these conditions and how one could lower the risk of dying from them.

1. Cancer

The Framingham Heart Study has shown that smoking and cancer are closely related. Smokers who quit can significantly reduce their risk of getting cancer. We also know that exercise and prophylactic supplements like fish oil and vitamin D3 have cancer preventative effects.

Antioxidant supplementation that included beta-carotene, vitamin A, vitamin C, and vitamin E daily or on alternate days for 1 to 12 years, along with selenium supplementation reduced the incidence of cancer of the esophagus, colon, pancreas, stomach or the liver. But bear in mind also that not all vitamins prevent cancer. Insulin resistance due to sugar and starch overconsumption is causing cancer, particularly breast cancer, colorectal cancer and endometrial cancer. I have discussed this in my blog "Sugar as a cause of cancer" (see references).

Pollution has been linked to increased lung cancer risks as discussed in another blog of mine (references).

2. Heart disease

Heart disease can be caused by several factors in combination. Lifestyle issues are important: Smokers need to quit smoking as the Framingham Heart Study has shown more than fifty years ago that smoking causes heart attacks. Obesity and diabetes also contribute significantly to the risk of heart disease. Often these are connected to faulty nutrition, which is another lifestyle issue that comes to mind when too much sugar and starchy foods are taken in; your liver will convert these into fatty acids, triglycerides and elevated, oxidized LDL cholesterol, which gets deposited under the lining of your arteries. A lack of exercise adds to this problem as a lack of exercise lowers the protective HDL cholesterol and fat is deposited under the lining of the arteries. Start exercising and your protective HDL cholesterol will rise. This means that your total cholesterol to HDL ratio will get into lower, healthier levels and you lower your risk for getting a heart attack. If you have diabetes, it is important that you manage your blood sugars well; this means that if you inject insulin, you want the blood sugar tests to be within the normal range and the hemoglobin A1C values to be well below 5.5%, which is the old upper limit; the new upper hemoglobin

A1C limit is 4.9%. As I mentioned earlier, Dr. Theodore Piliszek stated that the new normal range for hemoglobin A1C is 3.8 to 4.9%, quite a bit lower than what is normally recommended. Poorly controlled diabetes is an important cause of heart attacks and strokes. High blood pressure is also an important cause of developing heart attacks and strokes as well as heart failure. It is important to control your blood pressure by taking blood pressure lowering pills and also by exercising regularly. Exercise seems to send a signal to relax the blood vessels thus lowering the blood pressure, which in turn prevents heart attacks.

3. COPD/emphysema

Chronic obstructive pulmonary disease (COPD) or emphysema is mostly caused by chronic exposure to cigarette smoke from smoking. The earlier you can quit, the better your chances that your breathing will not be the limiting factor when you age. But it is also important to avoid exposure to other noxious gases, such as from welding and from exposure to pollution. This may involve a decision to move to a less polluted area. Or it might involve job retraining. Those who are suffering from COPD can be helped to a certain extent by a portable oxygen tank with nasal prongs.

4. Stroke

As mentioned before, quitting smoking, controlling high blood pressure, controlling blood sugar and exercising will all help in preventing strokes. If you suffer from diabetes blood sugar control is essential to stabilize your blood vessels including the ones that supply your brain. The key is to prevent hardening of the arteries by a healthy lifestyle. Exercising and keeping your weight under a body mass index of 25.0 have also been shown to be effective stroke prevention. Healthy nutrition as indicated above under "heart disease" is equally important for stroke prevention. Go green, eat more vegetables, consume more green smoothies, cut down grains, sugar and starchy foods, and you will live longer without strokes and heart attacks. Remember, what's good for your heart is good for your brain!

5. Unintentional accidents/injuries

Wearing helmets when bicycling, wearing seat belts when driving in a car, avoiding risky behaviors are all measures that save lives. One factor stands out in all of this: if you drink too much, you run the risk of being involved in unintentional accidents or injuries. People may not like to hear this, but your brain lacks the natural inhibitory impulses when you are under the influence of alcohol, so you become more daring and you may not pay attention to the split second that could have prevented an injury or accident. People react very differently to alcohol. Some people feel inebriated after only ½ a glass of wine or beer whereas others can drink more before they make mistakes. The best is to be sober. It is a law when you drive, but it is equally important when you ski, use power tools or walk in traffic. Even climbing stairs and ladders requires a clear mind!

Conclusion

As the CDC said 20 to 40% of premature deaths (deaths that occurred before the age of 80) could have been prevented, if the above-mentioned recommendations were followed. Let me rephrase this: 180,000 to 360,000 premature deaths every year in the US before the age of 80 could have been prevented! Curative medicine cannot help with these statistics. Heart attacks and strokes are merely an end result. Cancer and end stage lung disease are similar conditions indicating the end result of previously neglected prevention measures and now you are suddenly faced with this. And there are shocking, unintentional accidents that just seem to happen. This is where the importance of prevention can be seen. It is many small steps of prevention every day that are adding up to something formidable, a force to be reckoned with. Be part of the solution, think prevention!

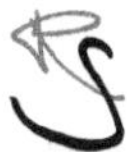

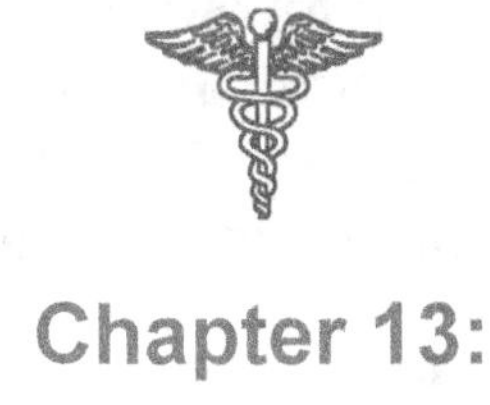

Chapter 13:

Supplements Yes, But Do Not Overdo It

The Dietary Supplement Health And Education Act of 1994 made it easier for people to acquire supplements and vitamins from health food stores. But since then there has been a proliferation of various products that are sold as supplements and not as drugs. It may give you the impression that all supplements are harmless, but this is not so. There are some supplements like vitamin A where you need to watch that you are not inadvertently overdosing, as toxicity is a problem; calcium supplements are also potentially toxic, if overdone. And amino acid supplements like protein supplements can lead to an overdose of brain hormones. Here is a sample of some of the supplements that may have side effects.

1. Vitamin A toxicity

Vitamin A is essential for normal night vision, for red blood cell production in the bone marrow and for the immune system. Under references you find a brief review about vitamin A metabolism. But while small amounts are beneficial for the body, high doses are toxic. In the 19th century the Arctic explorer Elisha Kane reported that consumption of polar bear liver caused severe headaches, drowsiness, irritability and vomiting within a few hours of ingesting it. It is now known to be due to "pseudotumor cerebri", a condition that mimics a brain tumor, but is caused by an acute overdose of vitamin A contained in liver as Shannon's textbook on poisoning and drug overdoses explains (see references).

In the US where people eat enough meat, fish and dairy products, there is no overt vitamin A deficiency. In Western countries there is a need to pay attention to avoid overdosing with vitamin A from multiple supplements. Simply read labels of any supplement you take, add up all of the vitamin A concentration you get and keep it below 5,000 IU per day. If you eat a lot of sweet potatoes or beef liver, do not supplement with vitamin A at all as you may otherwise overdose on this vitamin. Also keep in mind that a regular balanced diet including meat products has already about 5000 IU of vitamin A per day in it.

2. Vitamin C

Vitamin C is an important antioxidant vitamin and is needed as a co-factor for many metabolic reactions. It is participating in the production of collagen and connective tissues, helps with fatty acid transport and is necessary for the synthesis of neurotransmitters in the brain. The lack of vitamin C is known as scurvy; symptoms include bleeding gums from fragile capillaries, delay in wound healing and impaired bone metabolism. Although in the earlier research it was hoped that vitamin C would prevent colds and cure cancer, more recent reevaluations found that it does not prevent you from getting colds; it accelerates the recovery from colds by cutting down the recovery time by 25 to

30%, and it also does have some cancer protective effects. Higher doses seem to be more beneficial, but 1500 mg per day seems to now be the consensus of a reasonable upper dose limit per day for the regular adult consumer.

What about kidney stones? Several studies in the past have warned about vitamin C being broken down in some people into calcium oxalate kidney stones. Under references you find a brief Wikipedia review of the literature with regard to kidney stone formation. A study regarding the DASH diet, which is used for people with high blood pressure, showed that the incidence of kidney stones is almost half for both men and women compared to controls on a normal North American diet.

There has been a concern among the medical community that vitamin C as a supplement would increase kidney stones. However, a 2014 study showed that when both vitamin C and vitamin E are taken as supplements, the kidney stone formation goes down. Vitamin C does not cause kidney stones. This was one of those false rumors from the past.

Many inhabitants of industrialized countries including the population in the US and other countries are magnesium deficient, and this can be a major factor for forming calcium oxalate stones. But it has been known for decades that those who develop kidney stones excrete more oxalates in their urine, so-called "oxalate excreters". Under references you can find a 1996 study about oxalate excreters.

If you are taking in a lot of green smoothies from green leaf vegetables (spinach, kale, Swiss chard) that are high in water-soluble vitamins, you may not require any vitamin C supplements. In other words, think about how much vitamin C you consume in fresh fruit and vegetables. If you are consuming large amounts, be cautious about using additional Vitamin C. You should not exceed a total of 1500 mg to 2000 mg of vitamin C per day. Review your

family history: if any relative had a lot of problems with kidney stones, you may want to be cautious with vitamin C supplements, but most people do not have such a family history, they benefit from vitamin C supplementation.

3. Calcium supplements

Calcium is a key mineral in the body, important not only for healthy bone structure, but also to balance the electrolytes within the blood, in the extra cellular fluid space and within our cells. If calcium is low, the brain is more prone to seizures and the heart can produce dangerously irregular heart beats. We definitely need a balance of calcium! Because calcium is so central to our wellbeing, several factors work together to keep our calcium levels stable: the kidneys, the thyroid, the parathyroid glands, the adrenal glands, the bone as a reservoir of calcium, the gastrointestinal tract for absorption and a good, balanced nutrition. Dr. Rakel's textbook contains a chapter on "Vitamins and Minerals" where he points out that 4000 mg of calcium per day definitely causes toxicity. Where this becomes important to know is in postmenopausal women who supplement with calcium supplements for osteoporosis prevention: keep it to not more than 1000 mg of elemental calcium per day along with vitamin K2 (200 micrograms), vitamin D3 (5000 IU) and 500 mg of magnesium per day.

Absorption of calcium is dose dependent meaning that only 500 mg of calcium carbonate is absorbed at a time. Vitamin D3 deficiency reduces calcium absorption. But with high doses of vitamin D3, which is now often recommended, more calcium is absorbed, so it is important not to take too much of calcium supplements. They can also interfere with iron and zinc absorption, and when more than 2600 mg of calcium is taken, magnesium absorption is inhibited as well. Calcium can interfere with thyroid hormone supplements

(take 4 hours apart) and may reduce the effect of calcium channel blockers, drugs used for angina or high blood pressure. There is a balance between calcium stored in bone (99% of total body calcium) and the circulating portion of 1% of calcium in the blood. The parathyroid hormone and calcitonin are also involved in this balance. Hypercalcemia is the condition when calcium is too high. Common causes are the improper use of diuretics (thiazide diuretics), overuse of calcium carbonate supplementation, often used for osteoporosis, and overuse of vitamin D3, which increases the absorption of calcium. See your family doctor for blood tests and ask for advice how to supplement in your case.

4. High protein diets and protein (amino acid) supplements

Many protein supplements are available through health food stores and vitamin stores. The advertisers often state that our food would be substandard and these supplements would help "to regain strength". Athletes hope to get stronger muscles from amino acid supplements because they are the building block for protein that builds up muscles. Fact is that no supplements are needed when you eat balanced meals containing meat and fish and if you exercise regularly. The protein in your food will be broken down into amino acids and your body metabolizes this into to build up your own protein. I included a website under references that reviews the subject of supplementation with amino acids in sports minded people.

It is clear from this that we are dealing with a rather complex problem. Vegetarians and vegans may require these supplements to replace the missing protein intake. But the rest of us have to guard ourselves against overdosing with too much meat, amino acids supplements or protein supplements.

High protein diets (Atkins diet and others) have been glorified as being helpful for weight loss. But the long-term effect of high dietary protein intake leads to chronic kidney damage, in those with diabetes and high blood pressure as evidenced by protein leakage in the urine, called "microalbuminuria".

According to this reference the average protein requirement is 0.6 g of protein/kg body weight/day. This text comments that this would be compatible with the World Health Organization (WHO) recommendation for protein intake. For a person weighing 140 lbs. this translates into about 50 grams of protein per day. For additional information I have included a website under references that explains the upper limit of meat intake with the example of an 8-ounce portion of top sirloin steak.

Protein supplements have become very popular, but you need to be careful when you supplement with this that you do not get an overdose of amino acids. Amino acid profiling has been useful for physicians and naturopaths to examine deficiencies in children or adults checking for essential amino acids in the blood. However, in industrialized countries such as the US, Canada, Australia and others the larger concern is now the overuse of meat in our food (e.g. Atkins-like diets), protein and amino acid supplements. The same amino acid screening tests will find blood levels of amino acids in the toxic range that correspond to the composition of the amino acids in these protein or amino acid supplements. In this case it is imperative to stop the protein or amino acid supplements to prevent amino acid toxicity.

The safety of pre-workout supplements has not yet been thoroughly enough studied to know how performance-enhancing supplements affect the metabolism of the body (see under references). There are discussions that perhaps upper limits for amino acid supplements need to be established.

5. Creatine supplementation

Other supplements of concern are creatine supplementation in the sports-minded and in athletes who want to build up muscle mass. Creatine is synthesized by the liver from amino acids derived from fish and meat that is broken down into the amino acids arginine, glycine and methionine. There is no shortage in the food of industrialized countries, but athletes and sports minded people want to push the envelope and take in additional creatine that helps their energy metabolism in the muscles to increase their performance. Creatine is vital for the brain, the heart, the kidneys and the eyes (retina). It is a buffer for lactic acid during anaerobic exercise. Some of the side effects are muscle cramps, diarrhea, fluid retention and kidney failure when exposed to high heat and dehydration. Dr. DeLee warns in his 2009 Textbook of Orthopaedic Sports Medicine that there are no long-term studies of the use of creatine supplements, yet some athletes are taking them long-term.

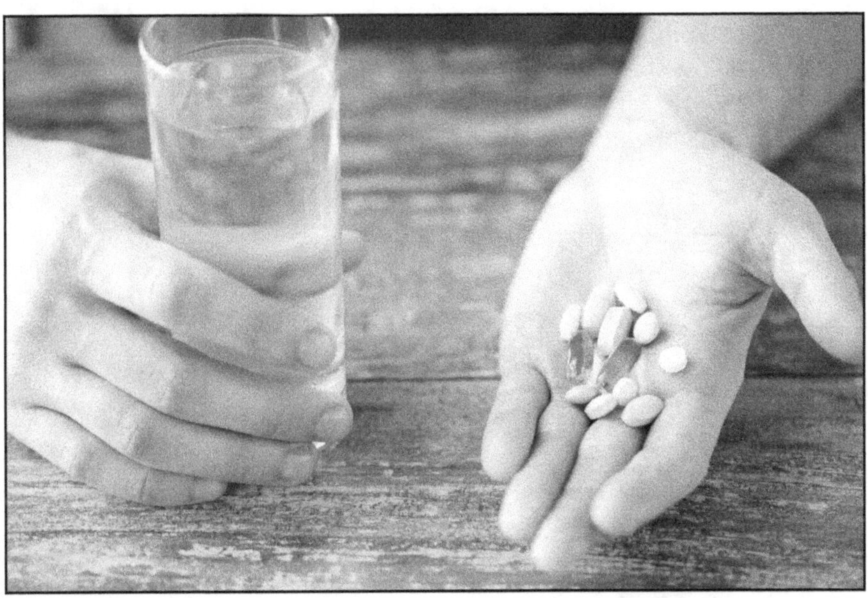

Conclusion

We are tempted by various merchants and infomercials to take in more and more vitamins and supplements including protein and amino acid supplements. But when you eat well-balanced meals, preferably organic food, you already have enough protein, nutrients, calcium, vitamin C and vitamin A contained in food. So you may be inadvertently putting a strain on your kidneys that have to eliminate whatever is too much for your body to take. Your liver may be quietly working overtime as well. Your brain gets overactive by the surplus of amino acids that are utilized by the brain to make brain hormones. Your system can only take so much; at one point a surplus of supplements will make you sick! It is important to be vigilant and think about what your regular food intake already provides. Do you really need that supplement or do you already get enough from your food intake? Are you falling for some marketing scheme? Remember, you are the steward of your own health!

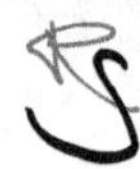

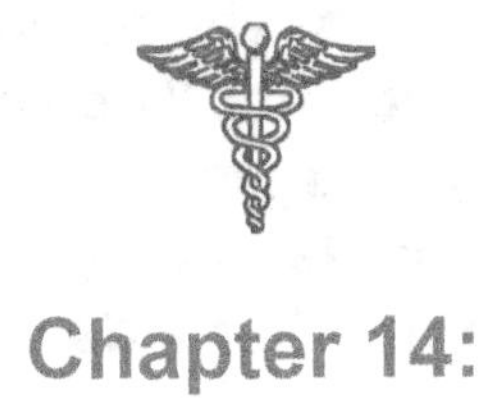

Chapter 14:

An Example of Alternative ADHD Treatment

When I think of the conventional treatment for attention deficit disorder, I am reminded of the history of medicine touched upon in chapter 1 when I described how patients or rather their symptoms were treated. Typically, a diagnosis is given, which often is merely based on the description of symptoms. Next a drug is given, which suppresses the symptoms. Essentially we are treating symptoms, but not doing anything about the cause. And this is what I will discuss in this section regarding ADHD.

Attention Deficit Hyperactivity Disorder (ADHD or ADD, attention deficit disorder) has been in the spotlight on and off over the years. What is hyperactivity? It affects 8% to 10% of school-aged children, and about 2% to 5% of adults who still have this condition.

Typically a parent receives a note from school that they must come to a teacher/parent meeting, and it is discussed that the child is disruptive in class, not paying attention, interrupting the teacher inappropriately and forgetting to do homework assignments. The teacher suggests that this may be a sign of hyperactivity. The school nurse is also of this opinion, and they suggest getting a prescription for Ritalin or Adderall (amphetamine type medications), drugs that have been shown in other kids to be fairly effective in treating the symptoms.

Next the doctor sees the child who confirms the diagnosis. A prescription for Ritalin (methylphenidate) is given.

In an attempt to quickly control the situation, the side effects of Ritalin are often not discussed in detail: agitation, insomnia, nervousness, anxiety, nausea, vomiting and loss of appetite, palpitations, dizziness, headaches, an increase in the heart rate, blood pressure elevation, and even psychosis as described in Dr. Ferri's Clinical Advisor textbook (see references).

It is easy to just write a prescription for Ritalin and hope that all will be well. Had the parents heard of all the possible side effects, they may have asked whether there were alternative treatments available. Even WebMD describes alternative treatments (see references).

The causes of hyperactivity (ADHD)

The exact cause of ADHD remains unknown, but there is a clustering of this condition in some families, and there seems to be a clear genetic component as Jacobson has described in 2001. It appears that several genes are involved, namely those associated with serotonin and glutamate transporters, but also those affecting dopamine metabolism. Males are affected with ADHD more often than females (in children 3:1, in adults 1:1).

Some remarks regarding brain development are in order: Dr. Kharrazian described in 2013 that the grey matter of the brain develops before the age of 9, and the development of the white matter is completed by the age of 19. In ADHD patients the frontal brain is underdeveloped, resulting in an inability to suppress unacceptable behavior, immediate desires and impulses. Prescription drugs may alter the behavior on the surface, but the frontal brain development is still lagging behind. The only thing that can influence this is behavioral/cognitive therapy and extra tutoring while the symptoms are controlled. The window of opportunity is closed by the time the ADHD patient has reached the age of 19. After that a juvenile ADHD turns into a permanent adult ADHD. The cases that had only childhood ADHD and outgrew it were the ones where the frontal lobe abnormalities had corrected themselves before the age of 19.

To complicate matters, the NIH has produced a review article showing that there is an association between a sugar and fat rich Western style diet and ADHD (see references).

Interestingly both Ferri, 2014 and Jacobson, 2001, which I would categorize as having originated from mainstream conventional medicine circles, deny such an association. But the 2012 NIH PubMed link also noted that a healthy diet with fiber, folate, and omega-3 fatty acids as well as supplementation with iron and zinc when these minerals are found to be low in the blood, do make a significant difference in ADHD patients towards normalization of their symptoms.

One of the under diagnosed causes of ADHD is gluten sensitivity as Dr. Perlmutter described in his book. This can spare the child or teenager the toxic side effects of anxiolytics, antidepressants or antipsychotics that may be inappropriately prescribed by their physicians. A gluten free diet would allow the brain to recover very quickly in such cases. A food sensitivity history and some simple gluten sensitivity blood screening tests will diagnose this condition.

To complicate matters even more, Dr. Amen has mentioned in several books that there are at least 7 different subcategories of ADHD that have been found in ADHD patients when studying thousands of single-photon emission computed tomography brain scans (SPECT brain scans). Dr. Amen labeled these as the combined type ADD, the primarily inattentive ADD subtype, overfocused ADD, temporal lobe ADD, limbic ADD, ring of fire ADD and trauma induced ADD. Dr. Amen explains that each of these types needs to be treated differently, and some of the treatment failures are explained by the fact that the treatment was inappropriate for the type of ADD present in the patient.

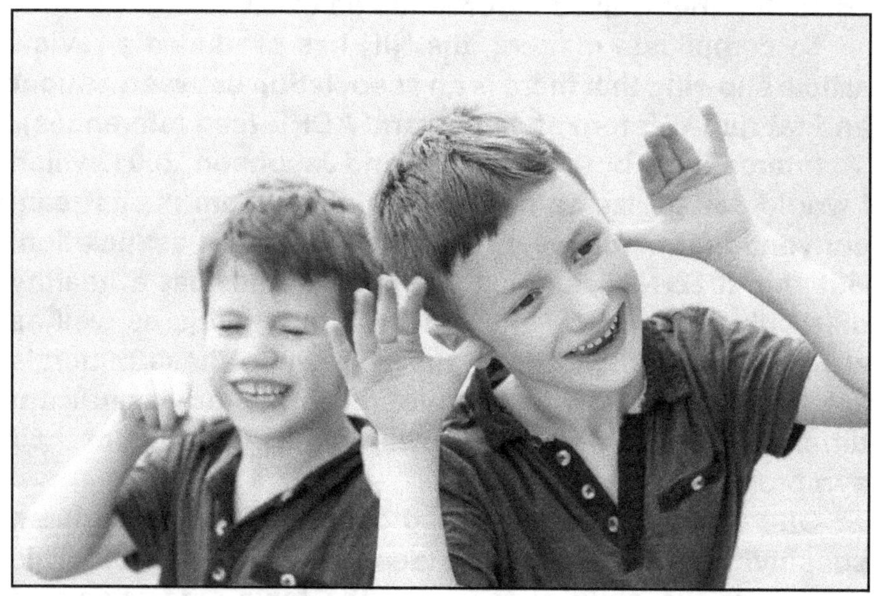

Treatment of ADHD

In the following I mention 5 steps that are useful for treating ADHD patients.

1. A first step toward normalization of the metabolic changes in the brain metabolism of the affected child or

adult is to adopt a diet that has been linked with low risk for ADHD: avoid food additives, cut out refined sugar, avoid foods that cause known reactions in sensitive persons. In other words pay attention to food allergies like gluten sensitivity and others. You may need to test the patient for food allergies using an elimination diet. Add a good amount of molecularly distilled omega-3 fatty acids, which is the pure form of omega-3 without mercury, lead or PCBs. This has shown beneficial effects in ADHD patients.

2. Involve a behavioral psychologist for behavioral/ cognitive therapy treatments. This is particularly effective in the 9 to 19 year old category where the frontal region of the brain is still developing.

3. Work together with the schoolteacher and get supplemental teaching in areas of academic weakness to reduce the frustrations in the classroom setting.

4. In adolescent girls who just started their period, a relative lack of progesterone (estrogen dominance) may be a contributory factor. A small dose (20 mg to 30 mg) of bioidentical progesterone from day 6 to 16 of the menstrual cycle may help significantly in alleviating the symptoms of ADHD. You will need to consult a naturopathic doctor or anti-aging physician to get a prescription for that.

5. If all of this helps only marginally, then a smaller amount of Ritalin may be helpful; however, blood tests should be drawn from time to time to monitor for drug toxicity as the rate of absorption and elimination of the drug varies significantly from patient to patient.

It is interesting that studies have shown that a combination of Ritalin or Adderall with alternative treatment methods had a better outcome than either method alone.

Conclusion

It is important to think about the various possible causes of ADHD and not just get caught up in the knee-jerk reflex of treating ADHD with Ritalin symptomatically. This is really only the last step, if everything else has not shown any benefit. Using alternative ways at home first, such as changing the diet, possible addition of low dose bioidentical progesterone cream in girls and co-operating with the school system with tutoring, the need for Ritalin may be avoided. If all else fails, the conservative approach is still available, but I suggest that drug monitoring (Ritalin blood levels) should be done from time to time. This will avoid Ritalin toxicity; blood level testing should be continued as long as this drug is taken.

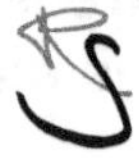

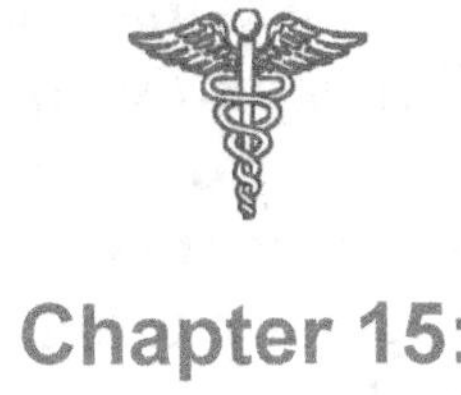

Chapter 15:

Summary

Throughout this book I have emphasized that we want to achieve a healthy, long lasting life through natural means as much as possible. Conventional medicine shines when it comes to laparoscopic surgeries, stents for clogged coronary arteries or complete joint replacements. But for chronic illnesses conventional medicine often fails, as explained with the treatment of famous people in chapter 1. Modern drugs often make the patient worse from side effects as explained in chapter 2. As shown in the book there are often alternatives available. A good solution is to combine the best of both worlds, which is called integrative medicine. If you can find an integrative medicine practitioner who does that, seek his or her advice.

We have seen that conventional medicine treats heart attacks, strokes, arthritis, high blood pressure and high cholesterol as separate entities. In reality these conditions start with wrong nutrition where too much sugar oxidizes LDL cholesterol, which aggressively undermines the normal lining of the arteries. This in turn leads to a loss of nitric oxide so that blood pressure gets elevated. All these negative changes eventually lead to heart attacks

and strokes. This process causes chronic inflammation, which also causes arthritis and with the breakdown of the immune system can also lead to cancer. To prevent this from happening we need to concentrate on good nutrition (Mediterranean diet), regular exercise and supplements to stabilize our mitochondria.

Cancer treatment will be completely revamped in the next years or decades. I have touched on this in chapter 10. Photodynamic therapy as described, using the Weber system from Germany and other newer technologies, will likely be the new standard. It is effective and has hardly any side effects. I suspect that some conventional oncologists will fight this till they are proven wrong.

I feel strongly about doing hormone tests early and replacing what is missing as explained in chapter 11. We are losing hormones as we age. The body is meant to be stable, and hormones are one of the stabilizing factors so taking hormones away with aging de-stabilizes our health. Take note that all our cells have hormone receptors, which need to be stimulated or our health will deteriorate. Melatonin is one of the hormones that fades away early on in life. Use melatonin to help you fall asleep. It is also a regulatory hormone that stabilizes other hormones. Later in life the thyroid often gets weak. Your blood tests will indicate this, and thyroid replacement with Armour (both T3 and T4) will rectify the deficiency. Finally, when you approach the change of life (women's menopause around 35 to 45, men's andropause around 50 to 60), hormones like DHEA, estradiol and progesterone in women and DHEA and testosterone in men will have to be measured and if low, get replaced.

As mentioned in the book, balanced nutrition with organic food, vitamins and supplements and exercise will all contribute to having optimal mitochondrial function that

results in lots of energy to enjoy life and stay active. All of this has been dealt with in chapter 7 (nutrition), chapter 13 (supplements and vitamins) and chapter 12 (general thoughts on anti-aging).

When you learn from "Healing Gone Wrong - Healing Done Right", you will experience successful healing and prevent major diseases from shortening your life. You will feel the power of prevention and avoid illness and disability. You are the one who is entitled to make the right choice!

Ray M. Schilling, MD
Kelowna, BC, Canada
January 2016

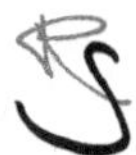

References

Chapter 1: Famous Patients Failed by Medicine

Elvis Presley:
Zittlau, Joerg (in German): "Matt und elend lag er da". Ullstein 2009

Wilson, James L., ND, DC, PhD: "Adrenal Fatigue, the 21sty Century Stress Syndrome - what is it and how you can recover"; Second printing 2002, Smart Publications.com

JFK:
Health and Medical History of President John kennedy: http://www.doctorzebra.com/prez/g35.htm

Churchill:
Zittlau, Joerg (in German): "Matt und elend lag er da". Ullstein 2009

Lord McMoran:
"Churchill at war 1940-1945". Robinson Publishing, October 24, 2002.
Beethoven:
Beethoven's medical illnesses:
http://www.lucare.com/immortal/med.html

Beethoven autopsy report:
http://www.awesomestories.com/assets/beethoven-autopsy-report

Lead poisoning of Beethoven:
http://www.lead.org.au/lanv8n3/lanv8n3-6.html

Michael Jackson:
Michael Jackson's health and appearance:
http://en.wikipedia.org/wiki/Michael_Jackson's_health_and_appearance

Michael Jackson autopsy report:
http://en.wikipedia.org/wiki/Death_of_Michael_Jackson#Autopsies

Chapter 2: How Modern Drugs Come and Go

"Epocrates" is a computer program for physicians that shows drug interactions:
http://www.epocrates.com/

What went wrong with VIOXX:
http://www.askdrray.com/what-went-wrong-with-vioxx/ (Oct. 2004).

Writing Group for the Women's Health Initiative Investigators: Risks and benefits of estrogen plus progestin in healthy postmenopausal women. Principal results from the Women's Health Initiative randomized controlled trial. JAMA 2002; 288:321-333.

Adrenergic receptor:
http://en.wikipedia.org/wiki/Adrenergic_receptor

Drug approval process:
http://www.alzheimer.ca/en/About-dementia/Treatment-options/Drugs-approved-for-Alzheimers-disease
Drug interaction concerning the cytochrome P 450 enzyme:
http://en.wikipedia.org/wiki/Erythromycin#Interactions

Chapter 3: Treating Symptoms Rather Than the Cause

Wilson, James L., ND, DC, PhD: "Adrenal Fatigue, the 21sty Century Stress Syndrome - what is it and how you can recover"; Second printing 2002, Smart Publications. com

Cytochrome P450: http://en.wikipedia.org/wiki/Cytochrome_P450

Chapter 4: Preventing Illness, Concept of Anti-Aging

Mitochondrion: http://en.wikipedia.org/wiki/Mitochondrion

Mutations in mitochondria: http://www.ncbi.nlm.nih.gov/pmc/articles/PMC147381/pdf/261268.pdf

Vitamins and supplements to support the body's metabolism: http://nethealthbook.com/health-nutrition-and-fitness/nutrition/vitamins-minerals-supplements/

Chapter 5: Keep a Healthy Brain

http://www.askdrray.com/preserve-your-memory/
The fact that statins can cause Alzheimer's is mentioned in: David Perlmutter, MD: "Grain Brain. The Surprising Truth About Wheat, Carbs, And Sugar-Your Brain's Silent Killers." Little, Brown and Company, New York, 2013.

Do not eat the "The Dirty Dozen" (Environmental Working Group):

http://www.ewg.org/foodnews/dirty_dozen_list.php

Avoid brain atrophy:

http://www.askdrray.com/avoid-brain-atrophy/

"Whatever is good for the heart, is good for the brain", from: David Perlmutter, MD: "Grain Brain. The Surprising Truth About Wheat, Carbs, And Sugar-Your Brain's Silent Killers." Little, Brown and Company, New York, 2013.

Jack de la Torre (2012):

http://www.ncbi.nlm.nih.gov/pmc/articles/PMC3518077/

William J. Walsh, PhD: "Nutrient Power. Heal your biochemistry and heal your brain". Skyhorse Publishing, 2014.

Rhode Island Hospital study regarding fish oil supplements:

http://www.ncbi.nlm.nih.gov/pubmed/24954371

Alcohol robs you of memory later in life:

http://www.askdrray.com/early-alcohol-use-will-result-in-memory-loss-later-in-life/

Review of the effects of alcohol: Kumar: Robbins and Cotran: Pathologic Basis of Disease, Professional Edition, 8th ed. © 2009 Saunders

Guardian news, 2014:

http://www.theguardian.com/world/2014/jan/31/russian-men-losing-years-to-vodka

Literature overview regarding protective effect of alcohol and effect of alcohol on atrial fibrillation and holiday heart described here: Bonow: Braunwald's Heart Disease – A Textbook of Cardiovascular Medicine, 9th ed. © 2011 Saunders

More information on alcoholism: http://nethealthbook.com/drug-addiction/alcoholism/

What alcohol does to you: http://www.askdrray.com/what-alcohol-does-to-you/

John T. Finnell: "Alcohol-Related Disease" Rosen's Emergency Medicine, Chapter 185, 2378-2394. Saunders 2014.

French paradox explained: "Hurst's The Heart", 13th edition, The McGraw-Hill Companies, Inc., 2011. Chapter 54. Coronary Blood Flow and Myocardial Ischemia.

WHO: Alcohol: http://www.who.int/substance_abuse/facts/alcohol/en/

Ivan Rusyn and Ramon Bataller: "Alcohol and toxicity", 2013-08-01Z, Volume 59, Issue 2, Pages 387-388; copyright 2013 European Association for the Study of the Liver

Regarding statistics on drinking in elderly: Tom J. Wachtel and Marsha D. Fretwell: Practical Guide to the Care of the Geriatric Patient, Third Edition, Copyright 2007 by Mosby.

Chapter 6: You Need a Healthy Heart

How to measure your heart function: http://www.askdrray.com/measuring-your-heart-function/

Dr. Steven Masley, MD: "The 30-day Heart Tune-Up – A Breakthrough Medical Plan to Prevent and Reverse Heart Disease", Center Street, A Division of Hachette Book Group Inc. New York, Boston, Nashville, USA © 2014.

More information on heart disease: http://nethealthbook.com/cardiovascular-disease/heart-disease/

Forget the low-fat diet: http://www.askdrray.com/low-fat-diet-not-protective-of-heart-attacks/

Lack of science behind the low fat diet guidelines: http://m.openheart.bmj.com/content/2/1/e000196

Senator McGovern's reply to Dr. Olson: http://www.docsopinion.com/2013/02/17/fat-and-heart-disease-exploring-the-villain/

Oiling of America: http://www.westonaprice.org/health-topics/the-oiling-of-america/#rise

High carb/low fat myth makes you sick: http://www.askdrray.com/buying-into-high-carb-low-fat-myth-makes-you-sick/
Framingham Heart Study: http://en.wikipedia.org/wiki/Framingham_Heart_Study

David Perlmutter, MD: "Grain Brain. The Surprising Truth About Wheat, Carbs, And Sugar-Your Brain's Silent Killers." Little, Brown and Company, New York, 2013. Study from the Netherlands on page 78.

Life Extension Book: Disease Prevention and Treatment, Fifth edition. 130 Evidence-Based Protocols to Combat the Diseases of Aging. © 2013

YouTube 2012, Dr. Ray Schilling: New approach to Medicine: How inflammation is the cause of many diseases:
https://www.youtube.com/watch?v=3X69pmVb3O8

William Davis, MD: "Wheat Belly Cookbook. 150 Recipes to Help You Lose the Wheat, Lose the Weight, and Find Your Path Back to Health". HarperCollins Publishers LTD., Toronto, Canada, 2012.

Dr.Schilling's book, March 2014, Amazon.com: "A Survivor's Guide To Successful Aging: With recipes for 1 week provided by Christina Schilling":
http://www.amazon.com/Survivors-Guide-Successful-Aging-Christina/dp/1494765330/ref=sr_1_1?ie=UTF8&qid=1398270215&sr=8-1&keywords=books+dr.+schilling

More information on: Arteriosclerosis:
http://nethealthbook.com/cardiovascular-disease/heart-disease/atherosclerosis-the-missing-link-between-strokes-and-heart-attacks/

Paradigm shift regarding hardening of the arteries: My book "A Survivor's Guide To Successful Aging: With recipes for 1 week provided by Christina Schilling" explains the content of this topic in much more detail.

Any kind of smoking is bad for you: Smoking still a health hazard:

http://www.askdrray.com/smoking-remains-a-health-hazard/

Who smokes in the US?

http://money.cnn.com/infographic/news/who-smokes-in-the-us/?hpt=hp_t3

Effect of smoking on different tissues: Mason: Murray and Nadel's Textbook of Respiratory Medicine, 5th ed.© 2010 Saunders

CDC Quit smoking resources:

http://www.cdc.gov/tobacco/quit_smoking/how_to_quit/resources/

More information on some of the topics mentioned:

Lung cancer and other cancers: http://nethealthbook.com/cancer-overview/overview/epidemiology-cancer-origin-reason-cancer/

Heart attack:

http://nethealthbook.com/cardiovascular-disease/heart-disease/heart-attack-myocardial-infarction-or-mi/

Chronic obstructive pulmonary disease:

http://nethealthbook.com/lung-disease/chronic-obstructive-pulmonary-disease-copd/

Smoking e-cigarettes of no benefit:

http://www.askdrray.com/smoking-e-cigarettes-of-no-benefit/

BCMA electronic cigarettes 2014:
http://www.bcmj.org/council-health-promotion/electronic-cigarettes-do-we-know-benefits-vs-risks

US Department of Health and Human Services. The health consequences of smoking – 50 years of progress: A report of the surgeon general. Atlanta, GA: Centers for Disease Control and Prevention and Health Promotion, Office on Smoking and Health, 2014:
http://ash.org/wp-content/uploads/2014/01/full-report.pdf

Chapter 7: Why Food Matters

B.J. Willcox, M.D., C. Willcox, Ph.D. and M. Suzuki, M.D.: "The Okinawa Program" Clarkson Potter / Publishers, 2001, New York.

B. Sears: "The top 100 zone foods". Regan Books, Harper Collins, 2001.

Ray Schilling, MD: "A Survivor's Guide to Successful Aging", Create Space, Philadelphia, 2014. Available through Amazon.com:
http://www.amazon.com/Survivors-Guide-Successful-Aging-Christina/dp/1494765330/ref=sr_1_1?ie=UTF8&qid=1398270215&sr=8-1&keywords=books+dr.+schilling

Holiday binges-eat now, repent later:
http://www.askdrray.com/regrets-following-holiday-foods/

Blog "My Peace of Food":
http://www.chicagonow.com/my-peace-of-food/2013/06/gallbladder-attacks-signs-symptoms-and-avoidance/

DASH diet:
http://www.nhlbi.nih.gov/health/health-topics/topics/dash/

"Thanksgiving dinner can be deadly":
https://suite.io/harriet-cooper/4e1b2fy

Gout leaflet:
http://www.patient.co.uk/health/gout-leaflet

Gout diet sheet:
http://www.patient.co.uk/health/gout-diet-sheet

Gluten sensitivity:
http://www.askdrray.com/gluten-intolerance-or-food-sensitivities/

Gluten-free consumer reports:
http://www.consumerreports.org/cro/magazine/2015/01/will-a-gluten-free-diet-really-make-you-healthier/index.htm

Rakel: Integrative Medicine, 3rd ed. Patrick J. Hanaway, MD: "Chapter40: Irritable Bowel Syndrome. Integrative Therapy". Copyright 2012 Saunders, An Imprint of Elsevier

Gluten sensitivity tests:
http://celiac.org/celiac-disease/diagnosing-celiac-disease/screening/

More information about gluten sensitivity:
http://nethealthbook.com/digestive-system-and-gastrointestinal-disorders/celiac-disease/

Sugar and starchy foods age you faster:
http://www.askdrray.com/the-problem-are-sugar-and-starchy-foods/

Dr. Ray Schilling: "A Survivor's Guide to Successful Aging". Paperback through Amazon.com, 2014:
http://www.amazon.com/Survivors-Guide-Successful-Aging-Christina/dp/1494765330/ref=sr_1_1?ie=UTF8&qid=1398270215&sr=8-1&keywords=books+dr.+schilling

Townsend: Sabiston Textbook of Surgery, 19th ed., Copyright 2012 Saunders

Melmed: Williams Textbook of Endocrinology, 12th ed., Copyright 2011 Saunders

More detail about how sugar from a high carb/low fat diet makes you sick:
http://www.askdrray.com/buying-into-high-carb-low-fat-myth-makes-you-sick/

More information on high density and low density carbs:
http://nethealthbook.com/health-nutrition-and-fitness/nutrition/carbohydrates/

Healthy sugar substitutes:
http://www.askdrray.com/yes-there-are-healthy-sugar-substitutes/

Blaylock: Aspartame:
http://dorway.com/doctors-speak-out/dr-blaylock/aspartame-msg-other-excitotoxins-the-hypothalamus/

More detail about how sugar from a high carb/low fat diet makes you sick:

http://www.askdrray.com/buying-into-high-carb-low-fat-myth-makes-you-sick/

More information on carbohydrates:

http://nethealthbook.com/health-nutrition-and-fitness/nutrition/carbohydrates/

Dr. Ray Schilling: "A Survivor's Guide to Successful Aging". Paperback through Amazon.com, 2014:

http://www.amazon.com/Survivors-Guide-Successful-Aging-Christina/dp/1494765330/ref=sr_1_1?ie=UTF8&qid=1398270215&sr=8-1&keywords=books+dr.+schilling

Soda study biased:

http://www.askdrray.com/industry-sponsored-diet-soda-study-deceptive/

Avoid restaurants or find an organic one:

http://www.askdrray.com/what-to-watch-out-for-in-restaurant-foods/

What is fat:

http://www.cdc.gov/diabetes/prevention/pdf/postcurriculum_session2.pdf

More information about: High blood pressure:

http://nethealthbook.com/cardiovascular-disease/high-blood-pressure-hypertension/

Cardiovascular disease:

http://nethealthbook.com/cardiovascular-disease/

Probiotics:
http://www.askdrray.com/probiotics-important-for-your-health/

Wikipedia: yogurt:
http://en.wikipedia.org/wiki/Yogurt

Bowel disease improves: PubMed 2013: Probiotics: http://www.ncbi.nlm.nih.gov/pubmed/23419530

Immune system booster: PubMed 2014:
http://www.ncbi.nlm.nih.gov/pubmed/24499072

Less respiratory infections: PubMed 2012:
http://www.ncbi.nlm.nih.gov/pubmed/22507276

Cancer prevention: PubMed 2014: Breast cancer: http://www.ncbi.nlm.nih.gov/pubmed/25114859

Probiotics help diabetes get better: PubMed 2012: Diabetes type 2:
http://www.ncbi.nlm.nih.gov/pubmed/22129852

Obesity: PubMed 2011:
http://www.ncbi.nlm.nih.gov/pubmed/20970896

Probiotics reduce cardiovascular risk: PubMed 2014: http://www.ncbi.nlm.nih.gov/pubmed/24330093

Olive oil: Study from Spain regarding lower mortality from heart attacks: PubMed 2012:
http://www.ncbi.nlm.nih.gov/pubmed/22648725

Increase in the more effective HDL2 particles from polyphenols, tested in humans: PubMed 2014:
http://www.ncbi.nlm.nih.gov/pubmed/25060792

Nitric oxide reference:
http://www.nutritionexpress.com/showarticle.aspx?articleid=286

Exercise produces nitric oxide: Bashore et al. 2015: Current Medical Diagnosis and Treatment 2015, chapter 10 Heart Disease. By Thomas M. Bashore, MD; Christopher B. Granger, MD; Kevin Jackson, MD; Manesh R. Patel, MD: Heart Disease. Lange, 2015.

4 months study on beneficial effect of olive oil: PubMed 2013:
http://www.ncbi.nlm.nih.gov/pubmed/22872323

Nitric oxide synthase:
http://en.wikipedia.org/wiki/Endothelial_NOS

Olive oil helps prevent heart attacks in metabolic syndrome: PubMed 2011:
http://www.ncbi.nlm.nih.gov/pubmed/21816783

Lowering blood pressure: Olive oil reduces need for antihypertensive medication: PubMed 2000:
http://www.ncbi.nlm.nih.gov/pubmed/10737284

Preventing heart attacks and strokes: Forbes: Spanish diet study:
http://www.forbes.com/sites/matthewherper/2013/02/25/what-to-eat-a-study-proves-a-diet-rich-in-olive-oil-or-nuts-can-prevent-heart-attacks-and-strokes/

Pure water:
http://www.askdrray.com/pure-water-a-necessity/

Toledo, Ohio incident affecting 400,000 residents: The weather.com 2014: Lake Erie:
http://www.weather.com/news/news/toledo-ohio-water-algae-lake-erie-20140802

BC toxic waste spill from a mining company's toxic wastewater reservoir, 2014:
http://www.canadians.org/media/recent-bc-toxic-waste-spill-alarming-unfortunately-not-surprising

Brief history of water purification: Sand filter:
http://en.wikipedia.org/wiki/History_of_water_filters#Sand_filter

Arsenic in soil:
http://en.wikipedia.org/wiki/Arsenic_contamination_of_groundwater

CDC: Water related diseases:
http://www.cdc.gov/healthywater/drinking/private/wells/diseases.html

Wikipedia: Walkerton incident:
http://en.wikipedia.org/wiki/Walkerton_E._coli_outbreak

Reverse osmosis:
http://espwaterproducts.com/about-reverse-osmosis.htm
CDC: Cryptosporidium:
http://www.cdc.gov/parasites/crypto/

More information on gastroenteritis (from unclean water):
http://nethealthbook.com/digestive-system-and-gastrointestinal-disorders/gastroenteritis-food-poisoning/

Food safety: http://www.askdrray.com/food-safety-crucial-in-summer/

Tropical storm Arthur: http://www.cbc.ca/news/canada/nova-scotia/food-safety-after-power-outages-when-in-doubt-toss-it-out-1.2698615

How is food poisoning caused? Chapter on food poisoning: Kliegman: Nelson Textbook of Pediatrics, 19th ed. Copyright 2011, Saunders.

Food poisoning: http://www.nhs.uk/Conditions/Food-poisoning/Pages/Causes.aspx

The “danger zone” for food in summer: http://www.homefoodsafety.org/food-poisoning/the-danger-zone

Treatment of traveler’s diarrhea: About fluoroquinolones: http://www.merckmanuals.com/professional/infectious-diseases/bacteria-and-antibacterial-drugs/fluoroquinolones

About trimethoprim/sulfamethoxazole:Wiki: Trimethoprim/sulfamethoxazole: http://en.wikipedia.org/wiki/Trimethoprim/sulfamethoxazole

More information on food safety: http://nethealthbook.com/health-nutrition-and-fitness/nutrition/food-safety/

Chapter 8: Healthy Limbs and Joints

Arthritis:
http://www.askdrray.com/stop-suffering-from-arthritis/

Dr. Mirkin's review of the Berlin study of Dan Dale Alexander's arthritis cure:
http://drmirkin.com/joints/1239.html

Dr. Kaufman's arthritis cure with mega doses of vitamin B3:
http://www.orthomolecularhealth.com/nutrients/vitamin-b3/

Dr. Frederick Klenner describes arthritis cure of vitamin C on page 76 and Dr. Hoffer on page 240: Andrew W. Saul, Ph.D.: "The Orthomolecular Treatment of Chronic Disease. 65 Experts on Therapeutic and Preventative Nutrition", Basic Health Publications, Laguna Beach, CA, 2014.

Dr. Hoffer: "Pandeficiency Disease", pages 24-30, a chapter in Andrew W. Saul's book: "The Orthomolecular Treatment of Chronic Disease. 65 Experts on Therapeutic and Preventative Nutrition", Basic Health Publications, Laguna Beach, CA, 2014.

Conventional treatment of arthritis:
http://nethealthbook.com/arthritis/osteoarthritis/treatment-osteoarthritis/

Osteoarthritis: change of diet:
http://www.whfoods.com/genpage.php?tname=disease&dbid=2

Dr. Schilling blog on laser therapy:
http://www.askdrray.com/laser-therapy-going-beyond-skin-deep/

Keep your muscles in older age:
http://www.askdrray.com/keep-your-muscles-in-older-age/

PubMed: Muscle mass index, 2014:
http://www.ncbi.nlm.nih.gov/pubmed/24561114

PubMed: Danish Study:
http://www.ncbi.nlm.nih.gov/pubmed/15292467

Falls and hip fractures:
http://shp.missouri.edu/vhct/case4007/index.htm

Stanford study:
http://www.dailymail.co.uk/health/article-105106/The-fittest-live-longer.html

Exercise in postmenopausal women:
http://www.maturitas.org/article/S0378-5122(14)00206-0/abstract

Osteoporosis prevention: exercise:
http://nof.org/exercise
NIH on life extension:
http://www.cancer.gov/newscenter/newsfromnci/2012/PhysicalActivityLifeExpectancy

Scales that work on the principle of bioelectrical impedance analysis:
http://jap.physiology.org/content/58/5/1565

More information on:

1. Exercise (fitness):
http://nethealthbook.com/health-nutrition-and-fitness/fitness/

2. Arteriosclerosis (hardening of the arteries and how to avoid it):
http://nethealthbook.com/cardiovascular-disease/heart-disease/atherosclerosis-the-missing-link-between-strokes-and-heart-attacks/

Prolotherapy and stem cell therapy:
http://www.askdrray.com/prolotherapy-and-stem-cell-therapy/

NIH introduction into stem cell basics:
http://stemcells.nih.gov/info/basics/Pages/Default.aspx

Details of interview with Dr. Reeves:
http://www.neurofascial.com/Interview

Platelet rich plasma:
http://www.elbowandhand.com/Patient%20Education%20Files/plateletrichplasma.html

Bone marrow aspiration:
http://www.aofas.org/footcaremd/treatments/Pages/Bone-Marrow-Aspirate-Concentrate.aspx

Liposuction:
http://cellbiomedgroup.com/technology/about-hampc/

Rotator cuff tear:
http://www.regenexx.com/2011/07/can-stem-cells-heal-a-retracted-rotator-cuff-tear/

Knee ligaments:
http://www.smartchoicestemcell.com/sports-injuries/knee/acl-injuries.aspx

Large disc bulge:
http://www.regenexx.com/2009/09/resolution-of-large-disc-bulgeherniation-with-stem-cells/

C. Everett Koop, MD, the former Surgeon General of the Untied States: A better way of life:
http://www.lifealert.org/koop.htm

Very small embryonic like stem cells (VSELs):
http://www.ncbi.nlm.nih.gov/pmc/articles/PMC2430762

Dr. Weber laser system:
http://www.dr-weber-laser-clinic.com/en/the-laser-therapy/the-principle/

Osteoarthritis of the knee:
http://www.mcrcindia.com/osteoarthritis-knee

FDA about stem cell therapy:
http://blogs.law.harvard.edu/billofhealth/2013/06/02/our-bodies-our-cells-fda-regulation-of-autologous-adult-stem-cell-therapies/

Knee with avascular necrosis:
http://www.regenexx.com/2011/01/knee-avn-osteonecrosis-helped-with-stem-cell-injection/

Chapter 9: Keep Toxins Out

Environmental toxins: http://www.askdrray.com/protecting-yourself-from-environmental-toxins/

The youngest and most vulnerable: Shannon: Haddad and Winchester's Clinical Management of Poisoning and Drug Overdose, 4th ed. © 2007 Saunders. Chapter 18:"Toxicologic Issues in the Neonate".

Diabetes from environmental toxins and risk from organic pollutants: Rakel: Integrative Medicine, 3rd ed. © 2012 Saunders. Chapter 31: "Insulin Resistance and the Metabolic Syndrome".

Volatile organic compounds and indoor air quality: http://www.epa.gov/iaq/voc.html

Cleaning product risks: http://www.berkeley.edu/news/media/releases/2006/05/22_householdchemicals.shtml

10 dangerous everyday things: http://home.howstuffworks.com/home-improvement/household-safety/tips/dangerous-home-products7.htm#page=1

Lead in jewelry: http://www.huffingtonpost.com/2012/07/17/lead-jewelry-california_n_1679683.html

How mercury gets into fish: https://www.whoi.edu/oceanus/feature/how-does-toxic-mercury-get-into-fish

Wiki: Marine pollution:
http://en.wikipedia.org/wiki/Marine_pollution

Radioactive pollution from Fukushima:
http://www.bbc.com/news/science-environment-23779560

Dr. John W. Apsley II : "Fukushima Meltdown & Modern Radiation: Protecting Ourselves and Our Future Generations", 2011. Temet Nosce Publications, Sammamish, WA 98075

Toxins in the bathroom:
http://www.askdrray.com/toxins-in-the-bathroom/

Get rid of toxins safely:
http://www.askdrray.com/get-rid-of-toxins-safely/

WebMD saying silver amalgam is safe:
http://www.webmd.com/oral-health/dental-health-faq?page=2#2

Living in a toxic world:
http://www.askdrray.com/living-in-a-toxic-world/

Vitamins, minerals and supplements:
http://nethealthbook.com/health-nutrition-and-fitness/nutrition/vitamins-minerals-supplements/

Xu, Qun, Parks, C.G., DeRoo, L.A., Cawthon, R.M., Sandler, D.P. and Chen, H. Multivitamin use and telomere length in women. American Journal of Clinical Nutrition 89 (April 2009):1857-63. Full text (PDF): http://ajcn.nutrition.org/content/89/6/1857.full?sid=9aab0e13-b4d2-42ad-b44c-15cffc6771c3

Wikipedia: Chernobyl disaster: http://en.wikipedia.org/wiki/Chernobyl_disaster

Mold allergies: http://www.askdrray.com/mold-allergies-often-overlooked/

Moldy dream home: http://www.jsonline.com/watchdog/pi/hidden-mold-in-dream-home-points-to-larger-industry-concern-b99178172z1-241158591.html

Hurricane Sandy: black mold: http://queens.brownstoner.com/2012/11/more-hurricane-sandy-aftereffects-do-not-mess-with-the-black-mold/

CDC: Mold after a disaster: http://www.bt.cdc.gov/disasters/mold/index.asp

Shannon: Haddad and Winchester's Clinical Management of Poisoning and Drug Overdose, 4th ed. Copyright 2007 Saunders

PubMed, 2005: Mold madness: http://www.ncbi.nlm.nih.gov/pubmed/15702814

More information about asthma: http://nethealthbook.com/lung-disease/asthma-introduction/

Lead still poisoning us: http://www.askdrray.com/lead-still-poisoning-us/

Are lipsticks dangerous?
http://www.cnn.com/2014/04/04/opinion/rasanayagam-lipstick-lead/index.html?hpt=hp_t4

Lipstick in the US:
http://en.wikipedia.org/wiki/Lipstick#United_States

Cosmetics for tribal ceremonies: PubMed, 2011: African children:
http://www.ncbi.nlm.nih.gov/pubmed/21665223

Kajal, a dangerous cosmetic: PubMed, 2010:
http://www.ncbi.nlm.nih.gov/pmc/articles/PMC3003848/

Pregnancy and toxins in Saudi Arabia: PubMed, 2010: http://www.ncbi.nlm.nih.gov/pubmed/21381557

European study about lead in lip products: PubMed, 2013:
http://www.ncbi.nlm.nih.gov/pubmed/23348610

FDA initiated lead study: PubMed, 2012:
http://www.ncbi.nlm.nih.gov/pubmed/23193690

Lead and chemical free lip products:
http://corneliadum.com/wpen/rouges-a-levres-et-gloss/

Shannon: Haddad and Winchester's Clinical Management of Poisoning and Drug Overdose, 4th ed. Chapter 73, "Lead" by Michael W. Shannon, MD, MPH, 2007, Saunders

Get rid of toxins safely:
http://www.askdrray.com/get-rid-of-toxins-safely/

More information on vitamins and detoxification:
http://nethealthbook.com/health-nutrition-and-fitness/nutrition/vitamins-minerals-supplements/

Implications of contamination with radioactive Cesium: http://www.ratical.org/radiation/Fukushima/StevenStarr.html

Protection from radioactivity:
http://www.askdrray.com/protect-yourself-from-radioactivity/

2014: More Fukushima spill:
http://www.weather.com/science/environment/news/fukushima-power-plant-leak-20140220

About Nagasaki and Dr. Akizuki 's team: Miraculously they survived:
http://www.washingtonsblog.com/2014/01/protect-radiation.html

PubMed, 2001: Miso soup saves mice:
http://www.ncbi.nlm.nih.gov/pubmed/11833659

Facts and figures about Chernobyl consequences : http://www.chernobyl-international.com/about-chernobyl/facts-and-figures

Q&A about Chernobyl:
http://www.greenfacts.org/en/chernobyl/l-3/2-health-effects-chernobyl.htm

Can it happen anywhere else?
http://www.hiroshimasyndrome.com/chernobyl.html

Wikipedia: Goiania accident:
http://en.wikipedia.org/wiki/Goi%C3%A2nia_accident

Cesium-137, a deadly hazard:
http://large.stanford.edu/courses/2012/ph241/wessells1/

Fukushima leak problems:
http://www.bbc.com/news/science-environment-23779560

Dr. John Apsley II: Radiation crises and antidotes:
http://www.drapsley.com/Pages/RadiationCrisesAntidote.aspx

Is it safe to eat the sushi?
http://www.theprovince.com/health/Fukushima+radiation+myths+experts+benefit+those+West+Coast/9401912/story.html

"The Implications of The Massive Contamination of Japan With Radioactive Cesium":
http://www.ratical.org/radiation/Fukushima/StevenStarr.html

More information on vitamins, minerals and supplements:
http://nethealthbook.com/health-nutrition-and-fitness/nutrition/vitamins-minerals-supplements/

Dr. John W. Apsley II : "Fukushima Meltdown & Modern Radiation: Protecting Ourselves and Our Future Generations" © 2011. Temet Nosce Publications, Sammamish, WA 98075

Update about the Fukushima fallout Water radioactivity 2015 much lower than expected:
http://www.hiroshimasyndrome.com/is-there-fukushima-radiation-on-north-america-s-coast.html

Fukushima video:
http://www.whoi.edu/CMER/news-and-events

Underwater nuclear weapons' tests:
http://www.ctbto.org/nuclear-testing/history-of-nuclear-testing/nuclear-testing-1945-today/

Akizuki diet reviewed here:
http://www.askdrray.com/protect-yourself-from-radioactivity/

Mediterranean diet linked to slower aging:
http://www.livescience.com/48983-mediterranean-diet-slower-aging-telomeres.html

Chelation for detoxification:
http://www.askdrray.com/tact-study-proves-effectiveness-of-chelation/

TACT study 2013:
http://jama.jamanetwork.com/article.aspx?articleid=1672238&resultClick=3 (J. American Medical Association, March 27, 2013, Vol. 309, No. 12)

Mayo Clinic results of TACT study:
http://www.mayoclinic.org/medical-professionals/clinical-updates/cardiovascular/results-trial-assess-chelation-therapy-tact-study-presented

Wikipedia: history of chelation therapy: http://en.wikipedia.org/wiki/Chelation_therapy#History

Heavy metal pollution: http://www.academicjournals.org/article/article1380209337_Duruibe%20et%20al.pdf

Organic food copper concern: https://www.extension.purdue.edu/extmedia/bp/bp-69-w.pdf

Zinc and copper in balance: http://drlwilson.com/articles/copper_toxicity_syndrome.htm#INTRO

Get rid of toxins safely: http://www.askdrray.com/get-rid-of-toxins-safely/

Living in a toxic world: http://www.askdrray.com/living-in-a-toxic-world/

More information about vitamins and detoxification: http://nethealthbook.com/health-nutrition-and-fitness/nutrition/vitamins-minerals-supplements/

Chapter 10: Reduce Impact from Cancer

Can cancer be beaten?
http://www.askdrray.com/can-cancer-be-beaten/
Wikipedia: Warburg effect:
http://en.wikipedia.org/wiki/Warburg_effect#Oncology

Þ. Lukðienë and P. De Witte: "Hypericin-based Photodynamic Therapy:I. Comparative Antitumor Activity and Uptake Studies in Ehrlich Ascite Tumor" Acta medica Lituanica. 2002. T. 9, Nr. 3, p. 195-199.

Here is another article by Dr. De Witte showing that phototherapy led to occlusion of tumor vessels by the combination of hypericin/photodynamic therapy:
http://www.bioone.org/doi/abs/10.1562/0031-8655%282002%29076%3C0509%3AATEBHM%3E2.0.CO%3B2

Michael Weber, MD: "New options of interstitial and intravenous laser therapy in oncology" The Intern.J. Med. Laser Applic. Vol1, July 2011, p.66

Chlorin E6:
http://www.webermedical.com/en/weber-medical-for-professionals/med-lasertherapy/photodynamic-tumour-therapy/

Curriculum vitae of Dr. Weber:
http://www.dr-weber-laser-clinic.com/en/dr-weber/dr-weber/

Laser therapy for pain:
http://www.askdrray.com/laser-therapy-going-beyond-skin-deep/

Michael Weber, MD: "Intravenous and interstitial photodynamic laser therapy: New options in oncology." To be published 2015.

Yellow laser:
http://www.webermedical.com/en/weber-medical-for-professionals/med-lasertherapy/the-new-yellow-laser/

Oxyven: YouTube: https://www.youtube.com/watch?v=qWRhxw9cH7U

Dr. von Ardenne: http://drsircus.com/medicine/dr-von-ardenne-on-cancer-inflammation-and-oxygen

Gemzar: http://www.webmd.com/drugs/2/drug-13449/gemzar-intravenous/details#

Xeloda: http://www.rxlist.com/xeloda-drug/clinical-pharmacology.htm

Dr. Hoffer: http://orthomolecular.org/history/hoffer/index.shtml

Dr. Hoffer cancer experiment with image of results: http://www.askdrray.com/can-cancer-be-beaten/

Andrew W. Saul, PhD: "The Orthomolecular Treatment of Chronic disease", Basic Health Publications Inc., Laguna Beach, CA 92651, 2014. Page 347 covers the Mayo Clinic "duplication" with only vitamin C, but not the rest of the Mega vitamins.

Lifestyle influences life expectancy: http://www.askdrray.com/life-expectancy-is-influenced-by-lifestyle/

Dr. Theodore Piliszek's talk: Methylation pathway: http://autismnti.com/images/Methylation_Pathway_Explained.pdf

Same:
http://en.wikipedia.org/wiki/S-Adenosyl_methionine

Wrong Hgb A1C recommendation in WebMD:
http://www.webmd.com/diabetes/guide/glycated-hemoglobin-test-hba1c

Wrong A1C recommendations from the National Diabetes Information Clearinghouse:
http://diabetes.niddk.nih.gov/dm/pubs/A1CTest/#6

Dr. George Rozakis' talk: Nutrigenomics:
http://www.genomebc.ca/education/articles/nutrigenomics/

Minor genetic errors:
http://genetics.thetech.org/ask/ask142

Different susceptibility to disease:
http://www.bbc.com/news/health-30021643

Telomere shortening:
http://learn.genetics.utah.edu/content/chromosomes/telomeres/

The methylation cycle:
http://www.dramyyasko.com/our-unique-approach/methylation-cycle/

Methylation and homocysteine:
http://www.foodforthebrain.org/alzheimers-prevention/methylation-and-homocysteine.aspx

Vitamin B complex:
http://www.dietitians.ca/Your-Health/Nutrition-A-Z/Vitamins/Functions-and-Food-Sources-of-Common-Vitamins.aspx

Migraine sufferers: http://ajcn.nutrition.org/content/85/5/1185.long

Defeat autism now: https://www.autismspeaks.org/resource/defeat-autism-now-project-autism-research-institute-39

Same: http://en.wikipedia.org/wiki/S-Adenosyl_methionine

Autoimmune disease: http://suzycohen.com/articles/methylation-problems/

L-methylfolate: https://www.psychologytoday.com/blog/the-integrationist/201310/depression-wont-go-away-folate-could-be-the-answer

Telomere testing: http://www.lifelength.com/pdf/Telomere-Measurements-in-Clinical-Medicine-Dr-David-Woynarowski-A4M-Orlando-May2014.pdf

Sugar can cause cancer: http://www.askdrray.com/sugar-as-a-cause-of-cancer/
Glycolysis: http://en.wikipedia.org/wiki/Glycolysis

May Clinic says "it's a myth that people with cancer should not eat sugar": http://www.mayoclinic.org/diseases-conditions/cancer/in-depth/cancer-causes/art-20044714?pg=2

Fruit fly cancer experiment: http://www.medpagetoday.com/Endocrinology/Obesity/40920

Sugar causes cancer:
http://www.jci.org/articles/view/63146

Three-dimensional cancer models:
http://www.ncbi.nlm.nih.gov/pubmed/17396127

Sugar promotes oncogenesis:
http://www.jci.org/articles/view/63146/figure/3

Low carb diet prevents cancer:
http://www.sciencedaily.com/releases/2011/06/11061411503 7.htm

Diabetes and cancer:
http://jnci.oxfordjournals.org/content/92/3/192.full

High glycemic load:
http://lpi.oregonstate.edu/mic/food-beverages/glycemic-index-glycemic-load

High starch linked to cancer:
http://www.foodnavigator.com/Science/High-starch-diet-linked-to-cancer

Harvard: Carbohydrates and blood sugar:
http://www.hsph.harvard.edu/nutritionsource/carbohydrates/carbohydrates-and-blood-sugar/

Wikipedia: Warburg hypothesis:
http://en.wikipedia.org/wiki/Warburg_hypothesis

Wikipedia: Women's' Health Initiative:
http://en.wikipedia.org/wiki/Women%27s_Health_Initiative

More information about hyperinsulinism that can cause breast cancer:

http://nethealthbook.com/cancer-overview/breast-cancer/causes-breast-cancer/

Sunburn prevention: The superpowers of vitamin D3: http://www.askdrray.com/the-super-powers-of-vitamin-d/

Tropical fern:

http://altmedicine.about.com/od/herbsupplementguide/a/Polypodium.htm

Life Extension: Protect against skin aging:

http://www.lef.org/magazine/2014/7/Protect-Against-Sun-Induced-Skin-Aging-From-The-Inside-Out/Page-01

WebMD: Sun protection:

http://www.webmd.com/skin-problems-and-treatments/tc/sunburn-prevention

More information on: Sunburns:

http://nethealthbook.com/dermatology-skin-disease/sunburns/

Different skin types and skin cancer causes:

http://nethealthbook.com/cancer-overview/skin-cancer/causes-skin-cancer/

When medical tradition fails - the unconventional cancer cure:

http://www.askdrray.com/multiple-myeloma-cured-with-measles-vaccine/

Canadian made modified smallpox vaccine virus: http://www.ctvnews.ca/canadian-made-virus-shows-promise-as-cancer-treatment-1.690978

Measles vaccine cures cancer:
http://time.com/103163/measles-vaccine-cures-woman-of-cancer/

PubMed, 2014: Prostate vaccines:
http://www.ncbi.nlm.nih.gov/pubmed/24838261

PubMed, 2013: Pancreatic cancer vaccine:
http://www.ncbi.nlm.nih.gov/pubmed/24498551

PubMed, 2013: Avoiding HPV immune escape:
http://www.ncbi.nlm.nih.gov/pubmed/23994536

PubMed, 2013: Brain tumor immunotherapy:
http://www.ncbi.nlm.nih.gov/pubmed/23302906

PubMed, 1974: BCG immunotherapy for melanoma:
http://www.ncbi.nlm.nih.gov/pmc/articles/PMC1344159/

PubMed, 2014: New type of melanoma vaccine:
http://www.ncbi.nlm.nih.gov/pubmed/24757523

Science Daily 2014: Genetically modified immune cells:
http://www.sciencedaily.com/releases/2014/05/140512124312.htm

People are not mice:
http://www.truth-out.org/news/item/23840-people-are-not-mice-the-failing-animal-research-paradigm-for-human-disease

More information on multiple myeloma:
http://nethealthbook.com/cancer-overview/bone-cancer/multiple-myeloma/

Vitamin D3 has super powers:
http://www.askdrray.com/the-super-powers-of-vitamin-d/

Low vitamin D3 north:
http://www.livescience.com/20910-vitamind-black-americans-cancer-disparity.html

Calcium, Vitamin D3 and Vitamin K2:
http://www.askdrray.com/calcium-vitamin-d3-and-vitamin-k2-needed-for-bone-health/

Defeat autism now doctor:
http://autism.about.com/od/alternativetreatmens/f/dandoc.htm

Swine flu:
http://www.sfgate.com/health/article/Flu-deaths-in-Bay-Area-rise-to-15-5141467.php

Dr. Cannell:
http://blog.litalee.com/2009/09/letter-on-vitamin-d3-and-h1h1-to-dr.html

WebMD: Vitamin D deficiency:
http://www.webmd.com/food-recipes/vitamin-d-deficiency

Live longer with vitamin D:
http://www.prweb.com/releases/2013/9/prweb11123378.htm

Vitamin D3 slows inflammation in MS patients:
http://www.nutraingredients.com/Research/Researchers-unlock-how-vitamin-D-may-benefit-people-with-multiple-sclerosis

Query vitamin D3 toxicity: http://www.webmd.com/osteoporosis/features/the-truth-about-vitamin-d-can-you-get-too-much-vitamin-

Safety of vitamin D3: http://ajcn.nutrition.org/content/86/3/645.long

Low calcium diet and corticosteroids: http://en.wikipedia.org/wiki/Hypervitaminosis_D

WebMD: The truth about vitamin D: http://www.webmd.com/osteoporosis/features/the-truth-about-vitamin-d-can-you-get-too-much-vitamin-d

More information on vitamin D3 for prevention of osteoporosis and hardening of arteries: http://www.askdrray.com/calcium-vitamin-d3-and-vitamin-k2-needed-for-bone-health/

McPherson: Henry's Clinical Diagnosis and Management by Laboratory Methods, 22nd ed., © 2011 Saunders

Rheumatic Diseases Clinics of North America – Volume 38, Issue 1 (February 2012) , © 2012 W. B. Saunders Company

Wang TJ, Pencina MJ, Booth SL, et al: Vitamin D deficiency and risk of cardiovascular disease. Circulation 117. (4): 503-511.2008. "Recognition and Management of Vitamin D Deficiency": American Family Physician – Volume 80, Issue 8 (October 2009), © 2009 American Academy of Family Physicians

Chapter 11: Stable Hormones Key to Health

Menopause:
http://www.askdrray.com/straight-talk-about-menopause/

Eileen Conaway, DO: Bioidentical hormones, 2010: http://abcnews.go.com/Health/womens-health-initiative-study-10-years/story?id=16397662

Predictors of menopause:
http://www.askdrray.com/menopause-and-perimenopause-in-women/

Dr. Lee: Saliva hormone tests:
http://www.johnleemd.com/store/saliva_serum.html

Calcium, Vitamin D3 and Vitamin K2:
http://www.askdrray.com/calcium-vitamin-d3-and-vitamin-k2-needed-for-bone-health/

Prevent heart attacks:
http://www.askdrray.com/two-approaches-to-heart-disease/

Melatonin is more than a sleeping-aid:
http://www.askdrray.com/melatonin-more-than-a-sleeping-aid/

The full story about testosterone:
http://www.askdrray.com/the-full-story-about-testosterone/

New England Journal, 2013 study about men:
http://www.nejm.org/doi/full/10.1056/NEJMoa1206168?query=featured_home&#t=articleDiscussion

Andropause when male hormone missing:
https://www.johnleemd.com/store/male_hormone.html

John R. Lee, MD: "Hormone Balance for men- what your doctor may not tell you about prostate health and natural hormone supplementation". 2003 by Hormones Etc.

George Gillson, MD, PhD, Tracy Marsden, BSc Pharm:
"You've Hit Menopause. Now What?" 2004 Rocky Mountain Analytical Corp. Chapter 9: Male Hormone Balance (p.118-148).

Randolph's website:
http://www.agelessandwellness.com/mens_hormone_health.html

How one man's life has been changed by testosterone replacement:
http://www.wpbf.com/health/hrt-not-just-a-womens-health-issue/25664954#!IIBrG

Bioidentical hormone replacement:
http://www.askdrray.com/bioidentical-hormone-replacement/

More information about male menopause (=andropause):
http://nethealthbook.com/hormones/hypogonadism/secondary-hypogonadism/male-menopause/

Dr.Schilling's book, March 2014, Amazon.com:
"A Survivor's Guide To Successful Aging: With recipes for 1 week provided by Christina Schilling":
http://www.amazon.com/Survivors-Guide-Successful-Aging-Christina/dp/1494765330/ref=sr_1_1?ie=UTF8&qid=1398270215&sr=8-1&keywords=books+dr.+schilling

Avoid burn-out:
http://www.askdrray.com/hormone-changes-with-burnout/

Dr. T. Hertoghe:
http://www.antiaging-systems.com/authors/36-hertoghe-md-thierry

Preventing burnout:
http://www.helpguide.org/articles/stress/preventing-burnout.htm

Adrenal gland disease:
http://www.uofmhealth.org/conditions-treatments/adrenal-disease

Low hormone levels:
http://psychology.jrank.org/pages/310/Hormones.html

Fludrocortisone:
http://www.webmd.com/drugs/2/drug-6802/fludrocortisone-oral/details

Depression:
http://www.rcpsych.ac.uk/healthadvice/problemsdisorders/depression.aspx

Hormone balance test:
http://www.johnleemd.com/store/resource_hormonetest.html

Chronic fatigue syndrome:
http://www.nhs.uk/conditions/Chronic-fatigue-syndrome/Pages/Introduction.aspx

Low testosterone:
http://www.everydayhealth.com/health-report/low-testosterone-guide/low-testosterone-fatigue.aspx

Lack of melatonin:
http://www.hatemeleishi.com/fordoctorspages/rheumatology/thevaguepatient.htm

PubMed, 2011: Adult growth hormone deficiency: http://www.ncbi.nlm.nih.gov/pmc/articles/PMC3183535/

PubMed, 2013: Overtraining (Adrenaline deficiency): http://www.ncbi.nlm.nih.gov/pmc/articles/PMC3648788/

Food cooked at low temperatures:
http://www.foodsafety.gov/keep/charts/mintemp.html

Common missing vitamins and minerals:
http://www.innerbody.com/nutrition/micronutrients

More info on adrenal fatigue:
http://nethealthbook.com/hormones/adrenal-gland-hormones/adrenal-fatigue/

Grumpiness:
http://www.askdrray.com/older-grumpy-people-have-higher-risk-of-dementia/

Finland study: grumpy old men and women: http://www.latimes.com/science/sciencenow/la-sci-sn-misanthropes-dementia-20140530-story.html

Grumpy old men testosterone deficient: http://www.dailymail.co.uk/femail/article-2532334/Should-grumpy-old-man-HRT-Despite-doctors-concerns-growing-numbers-men-insist-testosterone-jabs-transformed-lives.html

Symptoms associated with testosterone deficiency: http://www.theyucatantimes.com/2012/12/male-menopause-or-grumpy-old-man/

Sexual activity in various age groups reviewed in: Rakel: Textbook of Family Medicine, 8th ed., copyright 2011 Saunders

Women's Health Initiative, 2002: http://en.wikipedia.org/wiki/Women's_Health_Initiative

PubMed, 2009: The bioidentical hormone debate: http://www.ncbi.nlm.nih.gov/pubmed/19179815

Dr. Ray Schilling: "A Survivor's Guide to Successful Aging", Amazon.com, 2014 http://www.amazon.com/Survivors-Guide-Successful-Aging-Christina/dp/1494765330/ref=sr_1_1?ie=UTF8&qid=1398270215&sr=8-1&keywords=books+dr.+schilling

More information on male menopause (=andropause): http://nethealthbook.com/hormones/hypogonadism/secondary-hypogonadism/male-menopause/

Chapter 12: General thoughts on anti-aging

Mitochondrial DNA:
http://www.askdrray.com/frail-mitochondrial-dna-equals-frail-people/

PubMed, 2015: Less mitochondrial DNA associated with frailty and death:
http://www.ncbi.nlm.nih.gov/pubmed/25471480

Amount of mitochondrial DNA is what matters:
http://www.eurekalert.org/pub_releases/2014-12/jhm-aom121614.php

Tune up your mitochondria (Dr. Whitaker):
http://www.drwhitaker.com/3-ways-to-tune-up-your-mitochondria-and-enhance-energy/

2010 Life Extension Magazine about mitochondrial supplements:
http://www.lef.org/Magazine/2010/SS/Rejuvenate-Your-Cells-Growing-New-Mitochondria/Page-01

Stem cells/lifestyle/telomeres/hormones and stress
http://www.askdrray.com/stem-cells-telomeres-hormones-and-lifestyle/

Wikipedia: stem cells:
http://en.wikipedia.org/wiki/Stem_cell

Dr. McGinnis et al., 1993: Causes of death in the US:
https://galileo.seas.harvard.edu/images/material/2800/1140/McGinnis_ActualCausesofDeathintheUnitedStates.pdf

Wikipedia: telomere:
http://en.wikipedia.org/wiki/Telomere

Short telomeres mean higher heart attack risk:
http://www.bmj.com/content/349/bmj.g4227

Burnout: how to get back from it:
http://www.oprah.com/spirit/What-to-Do-When-Youre-Burned-Out-Consequences-of-Stress

Telomere length a telltale sign of aging:
http://www.askdrray.com/telomere-length-a-telltale-sign-of-aging/

Short telomeres mean higher heart attack risk (BMJ study from 2014):
http://www.bmj.com/content/349/bmj.g4227

More on lifestyle:
http://www.askdrray.com/lifestyle-has-profound-changes-on-our-system/

Dr. McGinnis et al., 1993: Causes of death in the US:
https://galileo.seas.harvard.edu/images/material/2800/1140/McGinnis_ActualCausesofDeathintheUnitedStates.pdf

Ford, 2009: Healthy living the best revenge:
http://www.ncbi.nlm.nih.gov/pubmed/19667296

Akkeson et al., 2014: Diet and lifestyle are what lowers heart attack rates:
http://content.onlinejacc.org/article.aspx?articleid=1909605

Michael Moss: Salt, sugar and fat:
at: http://www.amazon.com/Salt-Sugar-Fat-Giants-Hooked-ebook/dp/B00A1OZBSQ/ref=sr_1_1?s=books&ie=UTF8&qid=1418623366&sr=1-1&keywords=salt+sugar+fat+michael+moss#customerReviews

CDC obesity prevalence maps:
http://www.cdc.gov/obesity/data/prevalence-maps.html

CDC statistics of Canadian/US obesity rates:
http://www.cdc.gov/nchs/data/databriefs/db56.pdf

ABC fitness for kids:
http://www.davidkatzmd.com/docs/ABCManual.pdf

Dr. Katz: "kids speak YouTube":
https://www.youtube.com/watch?v=RnhzlVSQhSQ

Nutritional value rating system:
http://www.nuval.com/
2014 CoQ10 trial showing less mortality with congestive heart failure patients: http://heartfailure.onlinejacc.org/article.aspx?articleid=1911013

Blue zones in the US:
http://www.cbsnews.com/news/blue-zones-do-people-who-live-in-certain-areas-live-longer/

Focus on health:
http://www.askdrray.com/focus-on-health-rather-than-disease/
18 biggest problems with modern medicine:
http://www.care2.com/greenliving/18-biggest-problems-with-modern-medicine.html/1

Terry Wahls video:
https://www.youtube.com/watch?v=KLjgBLwH3Wc

Vitamins and supplements for MS:
http://www.healthline.com/health/multiple-sclerosis/going-herbal-vitamins-and-supplements-for-multiple-sclerosis

Wikipedia: H-2 antagonists:
http://en.wikipedia.org/wiki/H2_antagonist

Wikipedia: proton pump inhibitor:
http://en.wikipedia.org/wiki/Proton-pump_inhibitor

Licorice compound:
http://www.homemadehints.com/helicobacter-pylori-natural-remedies/

Wikipedia: Mastic gum:
http://en.wikipedia.org/wiki/Mastic_(plant_resin)#Medicinal_use

Irritable bowel syndrome:
http://news.harvard.edu/gazette/story/2010/12/placebos-work-%E2%80%94-even-without-deception/

The art of medicine:
http://www.npr.org/templates/story/story.php?storyId=129931999

Second part of problems with modern medicine:
http://www.care2.com/greenliving/18-biggest-problems-with-modern-medicine.html/2

Dr. Lee's website:
http://www.johnleemd.com/store/news_bhrt.html

TART trial:
http://www.nhlbi.nih.gov/news/press-releases/supplement/questions-and-answers-the-nih-trial-of-edta-chelation-therapy-for-coronary-heart-disease

Dr. Ray Schilling: "A Survivor's Guide to Successful Aging", Amazon.com, 2014, chapter 8, page 96.
http://www.amazon.com/Survivors-Guide-Successful-Aging-Christina/dp/1494765330/ref=sr_1_1?ie=UTF8&qid=1398270215&sr=8-1&keywords=books+dr.+schilling

Big Pharma drugs:
http://inspiyr.com/the-problem-with-western-medicine/

Prevent 40% of premature deaths:
http://www.askdrray.com/forty-percent-of-premature-deaths-can-be-prevented/

CDC states 40% of lives could be saved:
http://www.mnn.com/health/fitness-well-being/stories/healthy-choices-could-prevent-premature-death-up-to-40-of-the-time

Framingham Heart Study: smoking and cancer related: http://www.ncbi.nlm.nih.gov/pubmed/1845934

Not all vitamins prevent cancer:
http://www.askdrray.com/not-all-vitamins-prevent-cancer/

Sugar as a cause of cancer:
http://www.askdrray.com/sugar-as-a-cause-of-cancer/

Pollution causing lung cancer: http://www.askdrray.com/pollution-and-soaring-lung-cancer-rates/

Framingham Heart Study: http://www.ncbi.nlm.nih.gov/pmc/articles/PMC1449227/

Risk of obesity and diabetes: http://www.cnn.com/2014/05/07/health/time-avoid-dying/index.html?hpt=hp_t3

More information on: Cancer mortality: http://nethealthbook.com/cancer-overview/overview/cancer-mortality-rate/

Higher vitamin D3 intake lowers mortality from heart attacks, strokes, cancer, fractures due to osteoporosis: http://nethealthbook.com/news/higher-vitamin-d-levels-associated-lower-risk-mortality/

Chapter 13: Supplements Yes, But Do Not Overdo It

http://www.askdrray.com/overuse-of-supplements-can-create-health-risks/

Supplement Health Act, 1994: http://www.health.gov/dietsupp/ch1.htm

Vitamin A: Vitamin A metabolism: http://www.ebi.ac.uk/interpro/potm/2005_6/Page2.htm

Wikipedia: Elisha Kane, the explorer: http://en.wikipedia.org/wiki/Elisha_Kane

Shannon: Chapter 69: The Vitamins. Haddad and Winchester's Clinical Management of Poisoning and Drug Overdose, 4th ed.© 2007 Saunders

National Institutes of Health: vitamin A: http://ods.od.nih.gov/factsheets/VitaminA-Consumer/

Vitamin C: Mandell: "Water-Soluble Vitamins". Mandell, Douglas, and Bennett's Principles and Practice of Infectious Diseases, 7th ed. © 2009 Churchill Livingstone

Wikipedia: Kidney stone: http://en.wikipedia.org/wiki/Kidney_stone

PubMed, 2009: DASH diet kidney stone rate: http://www.ncbi.nlm.nih.gov/pubmed/19679672

PubMed. 2014: Take both vitamin C and vitamin E to prevent kidney stones: http://www.ncbi.nlm.nih.gov/pubmed/24460843

PubMed, 1996: Oxalate excreters: http://www.ncbi.nlm.nih.gov/pubmed/8770968

Calcium supplements: PubMed, 2010: Hypercalcemia and milk-alkali syndrome: http://www.ncbi.nlm.nih.gov/pubmed/20104639

Wikipedia: Calcitonin: http://en.wikipedia.org/wiki/Calcitonin

Rakel: Chapter "Disturbances in Calcium and Phosphate" and chapter entitled "Vitamins and Minerals". Textbook of Family Medicine, 8th ed. © 2011 Saunders

High protein diets and protein (amino acid) supplements: Review of amino acid supplementation: http://sportsci.org/jour/9901/rbk.html

"High Dietary Protein Intake" leads to microalbuminuria; in "Taal: Brenner and Rector's The Kidney", 9th ed., 2011 Saunders

Upper limit of meat intake: http://healthyeating.sfgate.com/many-grams-protein-eightounce-top-sirloin-8184.html

Wikipedia: Essential amino acids: http://en.wikipedia.org/wiki/Essential_amino_acid

PubMed, 2013: Safety of preworkout supplements: http://www.ncbi.nlm.nih.gov/pubmed/23515510

PubMed, 2012: Upper amino acid supplements: http://www.ncbi.nlm.nih.gov/pubmed/23077196 Creatine supplementation

DeLee: DeLee and Drez's Orthopaedic Sports Medicine, 3rd ed. © 2009 Saunders: http://www.amazon.com/DeLee-Drezs-Orthopaedic-Sports-Medicine/dp/141603143X

Chapter 14: An Example of Alternative ADHD Treatment

http://www.askdrray.com/alternative-treatment-of-hyperactivity-adhd/

What is hyperactivity?
http://kidshealth.org/kid/health_problems/learning_problem/adhdkid.html

Ferri: Ferri's Clinical Advisor 2014, 1st ed., © 2013 Mosby.

WebMD: ADHD, alternative treatments:
http://www.webmd.com/add-adhd/childhood-adhd/adhd-alternative-treatments

Jacobson: Psychiatric Secrets, 2nd ed., © 2001 Hanley and Belfus

Dr. Datis Kharrazian: "Why Isn't My Brain Working?" © 2013, Elephant Press, Carlsbad, CA 92011

PubMed, 2012: Western style diet:
http://www.ncbi.nlm.nih.gov/pubmed/22232312

David Perlmutter, MD: "Grain Brain. The Surprising Truth About Wheat, Carbohydrates, And Sugar-Your Brain's Silent Killers." Little, Brown and Company, New York, 2013. Look at pages 150-158 for ADHD and gluten sensitivity.

SPECT brain scans:
http://en.wikipedia.org/wiki/Single-photon_emission_computed_tomography

Daniel G. Amen: "Use Your Brain To Change Your Age" © 2012, Harmony Books, An imprint of Crown Publishing.
Nutritional intervention for ADHD:
http://www.ncbi.nlm.nih.gov/pubmed/21766545
Methylphenidate blood levels:
http://www.ncbi.nlm.nih.gov/pubmed/16958567

Combination of treatment methods for ADHD: http://www.additudemag.com/addnews/74/7639.html

More information about ADHD: http://nethealthbook.com/mental-illness-mental-disorders/developmental-disorders/attention-deficithyperactivity-disorder/

Index

B

C

D

E

F

G

N

O

P

R

S

www.ingramcontent.com/pod-product-compliance
Lightning Source LLC
Chambersburg PA
CBHW070219190526
45169CB00001B/23

9781523700905